Makeup is about self-confidence
and preservation as much as
beauty: getting you ready to face
the world looking your best.

To receive more makeup tips,
step-by-step tutorial videos,
as well as ideas on how to recreate
a more glamorous you, visit www.
glamournation.com.au

Makeup sequence photos were all taken and
retouched by Robert Bennett from ArbeePhoto
www.arbeephoto.smugmug.com

disclaimer:

My name is Jennifer Stepanik and I have been working in the makeup and beauty industry for over
fifteen years now. I have a very strong grounding in herbal medicine, having studied naturopathy,
and have qualified as a remedial massage therapist, reflexologist and reiki master. I then turned my
attention to the beauty and makeup industry and became a trainer in a spa, before starting my own
skin clinic, which I owned and operated for nine years.

I have over fifteen years of makeup and skin care industry experience and have written this E-book to
share my knowledge with others, so that everyone can add a touch of glamour to their lives and put
on their best face to greet the world each day.

While the greatest attention has been taken to provide accurate information in this E-book, it should
not replace your own research. Mature Makeup Application Made Simple is intended for information
purposes only and care should be taken when applying makeup to the eyes or if you have sensitive
skin.

TABLE OF CONTENTS

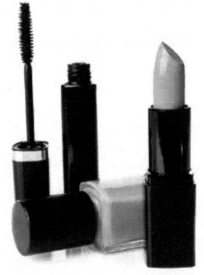

HISTORY OF MAKEUP

Augmenting our looks with a little powder and paint is nothing new, as women – and even men – have been using a wide range of products to enhance their features for centuries. Throughout the ages cosmetics have been variously associated with battle dress, religious rituals, tribal ceremonies, medicinal purposes, warding off evil and promoting good health, as well as to simply heighten beauty.

The beliefs and trends of the time dictate how society reacts, but while some critics say that modern women are under pressure to wear makeup, in fact it is only in recent years that we have had so much freedom and choice in the matter.

Ancient Egyptians used a variety of oils and creams to protect their skin against the harsh sun and drying winds, and they used many scents we are familiar with today to perfume their ointments such as chamomile, lavender and rosemary. By the fourth century BC, Egyptian women had created kohl from the sulphide of antimony or lead (later replaced by carbon or charcoal), which they used to define their eyes.

The driving forces behind Egyptian makeup were both medicinal and religious, rather than vanity, but a century later Grecian women succumbed to fashion by painting their faces with white lead, before applying a rouge of crushed mulberries and fake eyebrows made of oxen hair. Similarly, Chinese and Japanese citizens coloured their faces white with rice powder in a bid to conform to a trend.

Likewise, a pale complexion was sought after during Elizabethan England and so anything from organic egg whites to toxic lead paint was applied to the face to achieve Queen Elizabeth I's "Mask of Youth" look. Later, in the Renaissance, France and Italy emerged as leaders of cosmetic manufacturers in Europe and zinc oxide finally replaced the deadly mixture of lead and copper for face powder in the nineteenth century.

British Parliament passed a law in 1770 condemning the use of lipstick, with women who were found guilty of "seducing men into matrimony by a cosmetic means" being tried for witchcraft. Queen Victoria then publicly declared the use of makeup as vulgar and improper, reserved only for actors and prostitutes.

In the twentieth century, with the rise of ballet, theatre, television and film, makeup has become increasingly popular again. Indeed, during the Second World War, it was considered a patriotic duty for a woman to "put her face on" to look nice for the returning soldiers and maintain their morale. While the feminist backlash in the 1960s and 1970s rejected makeup as a sexist tool of oppression, fashion over-ruled such political statements as goths, glam rockers and new romantics alike used extensive makeup to express themselves.

Many commentators today suggest that modern society is obsessed with appearances, but this potted history demonstrates that we have always augmented our looks with cosmetics. More importantly, wearing makeup is now both accepted, but not expected – for the first time, wearing makeup is much more of a personal choice and a way of expressing ourselves. The contemporary trend of a natural, no-makeup look allows a woman to wear as much or as little makeup as she wants to suit her mood and the occasion. By subtly hiding any blemishes and highlighting positive features, you can allow your true beauty to shine through and give your self-confidence a boost.

Rather than feeling pressured into wearing makeup, most women nowadays invest a little time in their image and personal presentation by putting on their face, in the same way they would by styling their hair or choosing a suitable outfit. However, what looks good on us in our twenties, doesn't necessarily work for us as we grow older and so this E-book will help you understand how to flatter your features, rather than show up your imperfections, as you mature.

Whether you want a full going out look, or the bare minimum for every day, by learning how to put on your best face for your age, you can give yourself a lift and feel confident to tackle whatever challenges life brings.

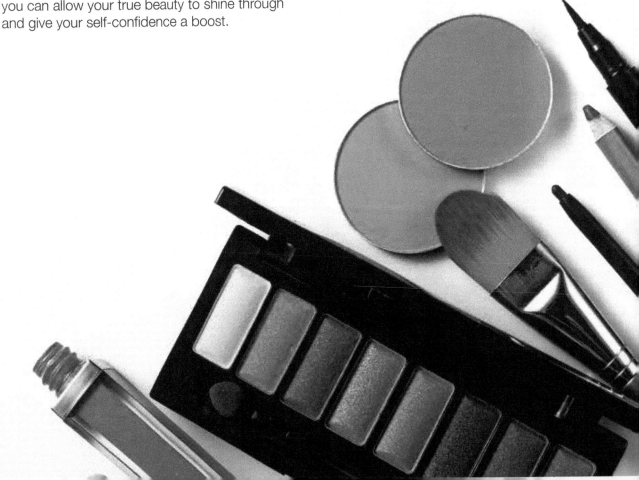

PREPARING YOUR SKIN

Your skin is the last line of defence to protect your body from outside forces, and so you can be forgiven for thinking it is tough enough to deal with the knocks of everyday life. But in fact, the complex number of functions performed by the skin, and the daily battering it receives from the elements, mean that it is very sensitive and any damage sustained is usually long-lasting.

Therefore, you should take good care of your skin at all times, but it becomes increasingly important as you grow older and your skin naturally deteriorates in quality. As you age, changes in your body affects the condition of your skin: menopause reduces the amounts of oestrogen and progesterone produced, while collagen and elastin levels decrease, both of which mean that your skin doesn't regenerate as quickly and makes it prone to wrinkles and sagging. In addition, the skin's natural production of hyaluronic acid and oil also drops, which leaves it feeling papery, thin and dry.

There are other, external, factors such as exposure to sun and cigarette smoke, which can prematurely affect the appearance of your skin. Conversely, eating healthily, maintaining good hydration by drinking 1.5 litres of water daily, exercising and getting enough sleep will help keep you looking young and vibrant.

By keeping your beauty regime as simple as possible you are more likely to maintain the habit, but there are a few key things that you should strive to do daily – cleanse, tone and moisturise with a SPF – as well as some weekly top ups such as exfoliation and facials.

The sooner you start a maintenance regime, preferably in your early 30s, the better you will look as you age, but it's never too late to start looking after your face.

If makeup is an art form, then your skin is the canvas upon which you will be creating your masterpiece. You want your canvas to be as clean and well-formed as possible, and there are ways of ensuring that your skin is primed and healthy before you start your makeup application.

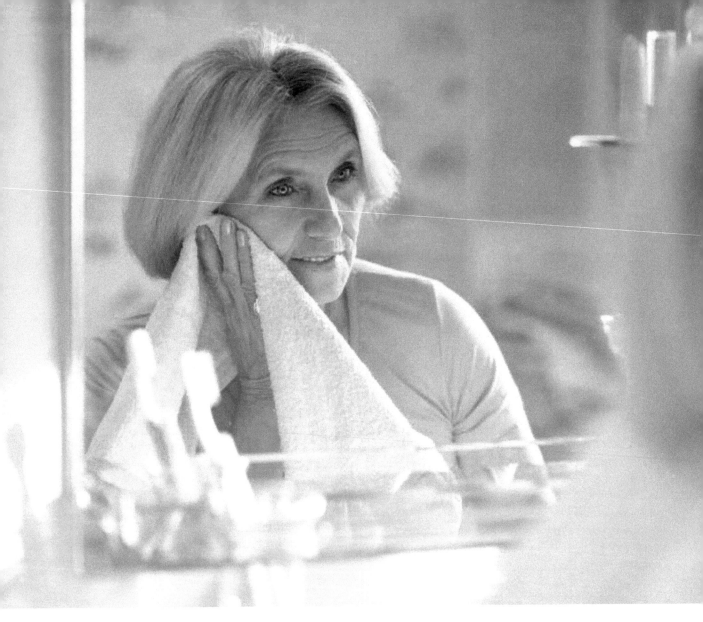

Step 1: Cleanse

To some it may sound obvious to clean your face first, but others may think it seems futile given that you're about to plaster it in makeup. However, if you want a good end result you need to start with a blank canvas, so the first thing to do is to clean your skin with an appropriate cleanser. The product you choose will depend on the type of skin you have and the feel you desire, but cleansing your skin twice a day will keep it looking fresh and healthy.

Aging skin tends to be thinner and more delicate and so you may prefer to use a non-soap cleanser, as soap can contain harsh detergents which strip away natural oils, leaving your skin dry and tight.

Gel cleansers

Suitable for someone who has skin that is prone to being oily. Gels don't leave any residue on the skin, but make sure that you don't use anything that's too harsh or it will deplete the skin's natural oils.

Creamier cleansers

Suitable for someone who has drier skin. Cream cleansers tend to leave a trace of oil on the skins and so are ideal for skin which tends to dry out, or most types during the winter to offer extra nourishment.

Milk cleansers

This is a lighter-weight facial wash; not as greasy as a cream cleanser but more soothing than a gel cleanser. Suitable for more sensitive and normal skin types.

Oil cleansers

It may sound like an oxymoron to clean your face with oil, but it works a treat because the oil in the cleanser attracts and dissolves the oil on your skin without removing the natural good oils. You don't need to spend a fortune in the shops as you probably already have the ingredients for the perfect skin cleanser in your kitchen cupboards.

Try blending castor oil with sweet almond oil on a ratio of 1 to 3 (25% / 75%). For oily skin, increase the castor oil to use 30%, with 70% sweet almond oil. For dry skin, decrease the castor oil to just 10% as it can be quite drying, with 90% sweet almond oil.

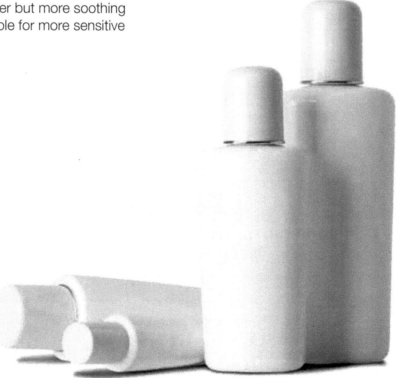

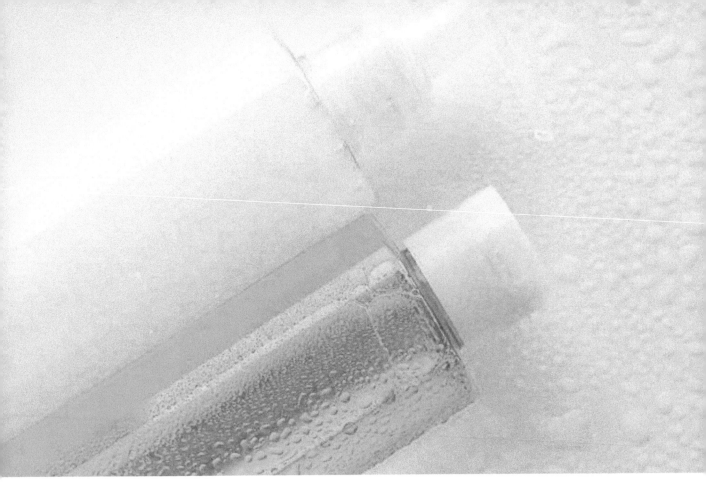

Step 2: Tone

Toners have always been marketed as a way of helping to restore the skin's pH balance after cleansing, however most modern toners are in fact like moisturisers and are predominantly used for nourishment and rehydration. They are packed with humectant ingredients which attract moisture to the skin and naturally hydrates and moisturises your skin.

You can either wipe a toner on to the skin with a cotton round, or spritz the toner onto your face holding the spray at about arm's length and keeping your eyes closed.

If you are looking for a commercial toner, choose one with ingredients such as Aloe Vera, which is not only hydrating, but also soothing and rich in antioxidants to help keep you looking youthful.

Alternately, you can create your own toner for daily use from equal parts Vegetable Glycerin and Rose Water. Simply mix and shake prior to applying to the skin and you'll have a beautifully soothing and hydrating toner for under $10. If you want more tips like this, visit **www.glamournation.com.au**

Step 3: Moisturise

It's a common misconception that you don't need a moisturiser if you have greasy or oily skin, but you need to replenish the natural moisture that has been removed, either through washing or by external elements.

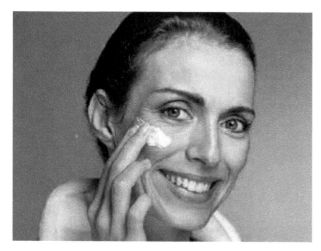

Like toners, moisturisers contain a combination of humectants, ceramides and emollients which attract moisture to the skin and trap existing water in the pores allowing the damaged outer layer of the skin the chance to repair.

Moisturiser Ingredients

Humectants - draw water to the skin cells to keep them hydrated, and are suitable for all skin types including oily skin as they provides a natural layer of moisture.

Emollients - fill in any gaps between skin cells, giving the appearance of a smoother surface and therefore are suitable for more mature skin which might have wrinkles.

Ceramides - help to hold the skin together and retain moisture, and they are suitable for normal or combination skin types, or those prone to eczema.

Occlusives - are super-hydrants and are more commonly used for body moisturisers, not the face, as they can be heavy and clog up the pores.

Types of skin

Oily skin - you should seek a light, oil-free, water-based lotion which will not clog your pores, but remember you do need to use a moisturiser.

Dry skin - you should opt for a heavier, oil-based cream and consider re-applying throughout the day if your skin is prone to cracking or flaking, or feels tight.

Combination skin - you should use an oil-based, cream moisturiser when the skin is completely dry.

Normal skin - you should choose a light, non-greasy water-based moisturiser for all round hydration.

Sensitive skin - you should search for a moisturiser without fragrance or colour, with a high SPF to prevent irritating your skin with the sun's UV rays.

If you are seeing the effects of time on your face, then try a moisturiser with anti-ageing ingredients such as Vitamin A, Vitamin E, Vitamin F, antioxidants, oils such as olive, macademia nut, avocado or grape seed, and essential oils such as rosewood, sandalwood, patchouli, geranium, lavender and rosemary.

Step 4: Exfoliate

You only need to exfoliate your skin once a week, but making sure you do it really well becomes increasingly important as you start to age. Dead skin cells naturally accumulate on your skin, clogging up the pores beneath them, but as you get older your skin cells regenerate at a much slower rate. Unless you stimulate the process by exfoliating, your skin will appear dull, uneven, pigmented and flaky. Regular exfoliation will give you a smoother, more even and brighter complexion and give you a better base to hold your makeup.

Almond Meal Exfoliant

Almonds are exceptionally rich in vitamin E, which is essential to repairing skin damage, as well as vitamin D, essential fatty acids, calcium, magnesium and potassium. You can benefit by using almond oil in a home-made cleanser, but almond meal makes an excellent natural abrasive substance which provides a great base for an exfoliating facial scrub.

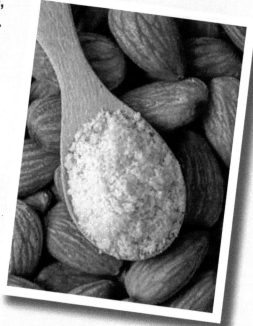

1. In a small clean bowl, mix 2 tablespoons of almond meal to 1 tablespoon of water with a spoon.
2. Wash your face as normal with your preferred cleanser.
3. Apply the scrub in a circular motion taking care to avoid the eyes.
4. Concentrate on the T-zone of the forehead, nose and chin.
5. Wash the scrub off by splashing water over the face. Don't wipe the scrub off otherwise you can pull at the delicate skin.
6. Pat the face dry and apply your preferred moisturiser.

You can replace the water with milk for a more moisturising version which is better for drier, more mature skin. The lactic acid in the milk has both a hydrating and brightening effect on the skin, which is combined with the emollient effect of the oil from the almonds to give you super soft skin.

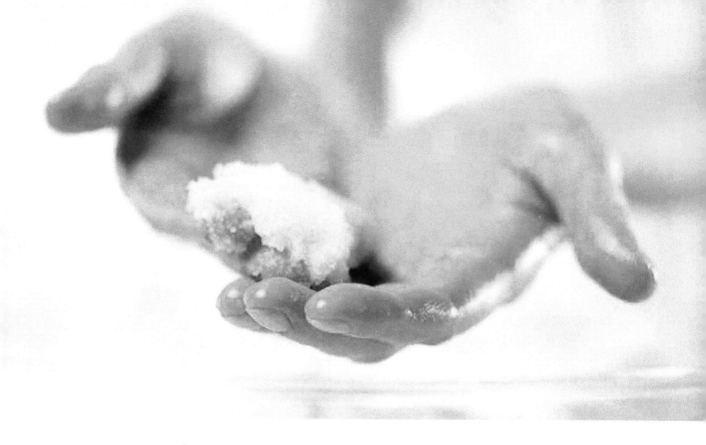

Types of exfoliants

Chemical exfoliants – these acid-based chemical peels often contain alpha-hydroxy acid (AHA) or beta-hydroxy acid (BHA) and can be quite harsh to the skin. They can be effective to reduce wrinkles, stimulate the production of collagen and plump up the skin, but can also cause sensitivity to the sun, or leave the skin temporarily red and itchy, so they should be used infrequently.

If you want to use a chemical exfoliant, choose an AHA one for sun-damaged or dry skin as they offer a lighter cleanse and improve the skin's hydration. BHA products should be used for oily or acne-prone skin as they offer a deeper cleanse to unclog the pores.

Enzyme exfoliants – these exfoliants work in a similar way to a chemical peel, but the active ingredient is a plant-based enzyme such as papaya, pineapple or pumpkin, and so they are kinder to your skin.

Physical Scrubs – these scrubs contain beads or natural abrasive substances to slough away the dead skin cells, the advantage being that you can literally feel the scrub working to revive your skin.

Fine sugar scrubs should be used for sensitive or dry skin, while oily skin can tolerate coarser sugar or the extremely abrasive microdermabrasion crystals. These scrubs can either be bought or made quite simply at home – for more information on the benefits of making your own sugar scrubs, please see **https://www.createspace.com/4383040**

Step 5: Facial

A professional facial is not only a time for you to relax and enjoy some personal pampering, but also an opportunity for you to give your face an overhaul. A good facial will cleanse your skin, stimulate circulation and improve the muscle tone, leaving your skin looking brighter, more even and feeling silky soft.

If you can't afford to have a regular professional pamper, you can give yourself a mini facial whenever you cleanse, moisturise or exfoliate your skin. Use the pads of your fingers to massage your face in a circular motion across your forehead, down your temples to your cheeks, along the side of your nose and across your chin. Be careful not to drag the delicate skin around your eyes, where you should only pat cream. You can finish with some gentle pinching and tapping movements to stimulate the skin and bring natural colour to your face.

Step 6: Prime

Once you have completed your cleaning regime, you are ready to start applying makeup. Many women prefer to start with a primer which creates a barrier between the skin and makeup. It can even out skin tone and provide a smooth surface on which makeup can be applied more easily. Primers also make it easier to apply foundation and help your makeup stay on longer. If you have enlarged pores you should apply this product with a latex sponge and really push it into the skin to create a smooth base for your makeup.

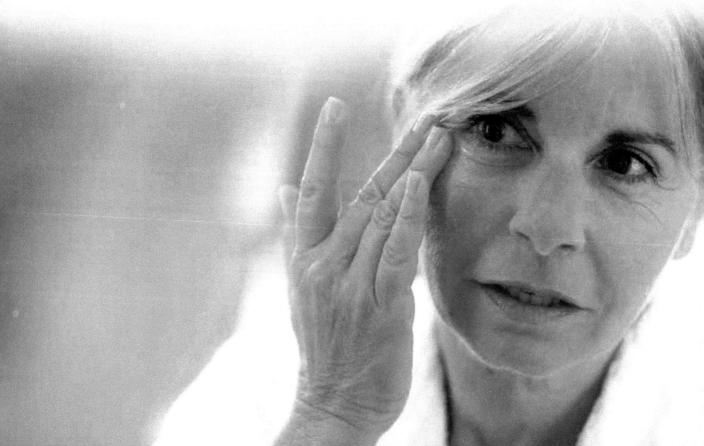

MAKEUP

Having prepared your skin, you need to first understand the different types of makeup before you learn how to apply it.

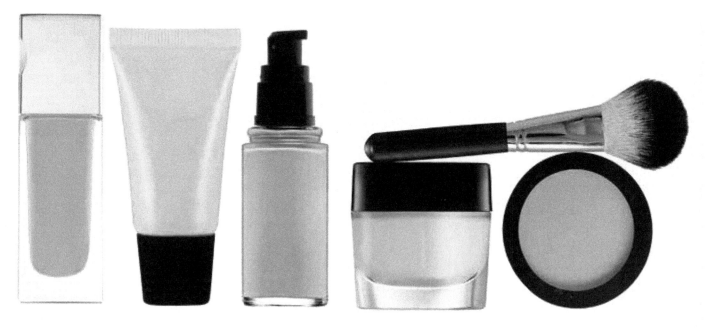

Foundation

The right shade of foundation will disappear into your skin, giving the illusion of not wearing any makeup at all, while subtly hiding any blemishes and leaving you with flawless-looking skin. Many women find they use two shades of foundation throughout the year – a paler one for winter and a darker one for summer to coincide with your naturally changing skin colour. You can apply foundation using a foam sponge, fingers or foundation brush depending on the type you choose.

Liquid or Cream Foundation

Liquid foundations are best applied by building up each layer, letting it dry between each one. People with oily skin sometimes complain that liquid foundation slides off a greasy face, and certainly the heavier cream foundations are formulated for drier, more mature skin.

Oil-based Foundation

This option is particularly good for someone with dry skin with some fine lines and wrinkles as the added moisture in the product temporarily plumps up the skin.

Tinted Moisturiser

Also known as sheer foundation, this product acts as both a moisturiser and a light foundation at the same time, but it won't do more than provide a sheer all-over cover so would not work for someone with very uneven skin.

Matte Foundation

Specially formulated for women with oily skin, matte foundation is also known as oil-free makeup. As it is drier than normal makeup and you need to blend it in as you apply it, so it works best on an extra layer of moisturiser or a primer.

Mousse Foundation

Also known as whipped foundation, it is liquid makeup which is made lighter and smoother by being whipped with air. It is suitable for all skin types, but is particularly good for dry or more mature skin as it glides on smoothly.

Powder Foundation

Also known as a compact because of its appearance, powder foundation is useful to have in the handbag for top ups during the day, particularly for women with oily skin who want to hide the shine. It can also be used to set liquid foundation and help hold it in place.

Cream-to-Powder Compact Foundations

Applied like a powder using a sponge and building up in layers, these hybrid foundations combine the matte finish of a powder with the silkiness of a cream. Coverage is light if you only apply one layer, or can be built up to full cover if preferred.

Stick Foundation

Essentially this is cream-to-powder foundation in a convenient stick form. This makeup is heavier than liquid foundation and can be prone to caking on dry skin, so it is more suitable for normal to oily skin. The thicker coverage makes it suitable for covering up any blemishes or scars. This type of foundation is easily portable and mess-free for popping into a handbag.

Mineral Foundation

Loose or pressed powder makeup, made primarily from minerals, this natural organic foundation is particularly suitable for someone with sensitive skin and allergies.

With all the above options available, don't be tempted into buying foundations that boast they can control and correct oil production as these claims are usually unsubstantiated. Likewise avoid foundations that purport to adjust skin tone or be colour-correcting, as neither results are satisfactory and do not justify the additional expense. It is much better to learn how to apply the right colour foundation correctly than try and cut corners.

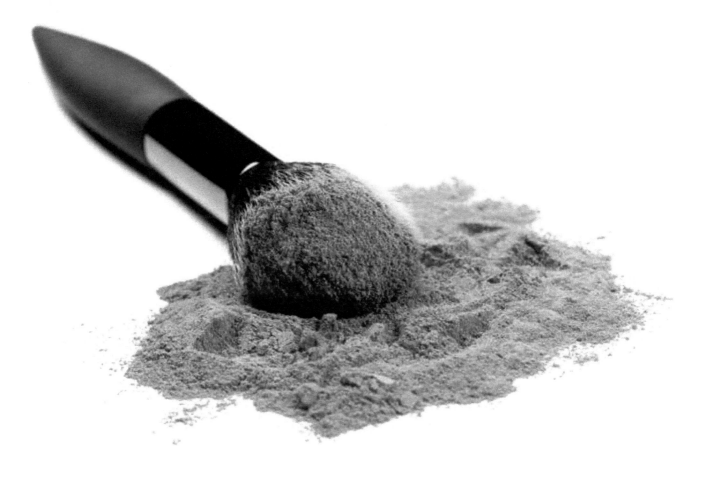

Eye Shadow

Eye shadow is a colour which can be added to the eye socket, brow bone and even under the lower lash line according to the desired look.

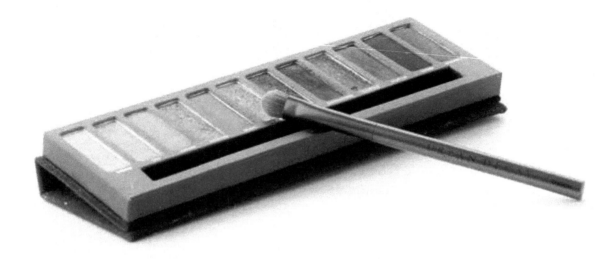

Powder eye shadow

The most common form of eye shadow is pressed powder which can be applied to the eye area using a makeup brush, sponge or even finger. But eye shadow also comes in loose powder form, although this can be messier to apply as the product can fall onto the cheek.

Liquid eye shadow

Looking like a lip gloss, liquid eye shadows come with their own built in applicator. Providing long-lasting colour, the downside is that the colour is not as easily blended. The liquid can vary in consistency between brands, so shop around to find a product that suits you and remember that it will have a shorter shelf life than powders.

Cream or gel eye shadow

A hybrid of powder and liquid eye shadows, these products still have a shorter shelf life and don't blend as well as powder, but have the staying power of liquid option. Typically emollient based, these eye shadows are very hydrating to the skin and feel smooth.

Stick or crayon eye shadow

Essentially these are cream eye shadows in a stick form which makes them very easy to apply and convenient to put in a handbag.

Eyeliner

Eyeliner is one of the oldest forms of makeup and is still going strong today. It is used to define the lash line on both the top and bottom eyelashes, and some can also be used on the inside of the lower lid, the waterline.

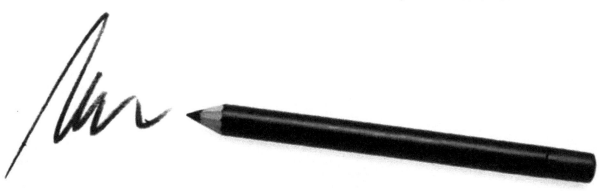

Eyeliner Pencil

Traditional eyeliner pencils are comfortable to use and provide rich consistent colour, either in a precise line after sharpening, or with a softer look when allowed to blunt slightly.

Liquid Eyeliner

Liquid eyeliners provide a bold slick look as the product is dispensed from a tube through a fine brush. You will need a steady hand as it can be quite tricky to apply and not very forgiving if you go wrong, but it is great for dramatic applications.

Gel Eyeliner

This eyeliner is creamier than liquid versions and glides easily, but will take longer to dry than liquid eyeliners and can easily be smudged, either on purpose or by mistake. As such, it can also be used as a base for eye shadows.

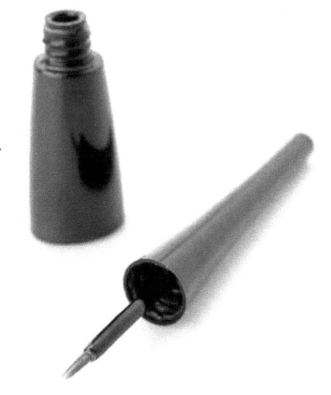

Eye shadow as Eyeliner

With a stiff pencil brush, you can use eye shadow as an eyeliner to draw a thick line along your lashes. The benefit of this method is that it can provide a subtle daytime look which can easily be augmented for an evening look. You cannot use eye shadow as an eyeliner for your lower waterline as it will irritate your eyes and will not hold.

Take extra care of eyeliner products as you can risk transferring bacteria to the eye and getting an infection. If you have used any products while you have had an eye infection, you will need to throw out the items and restock otherwise you will risk a repeat infection.

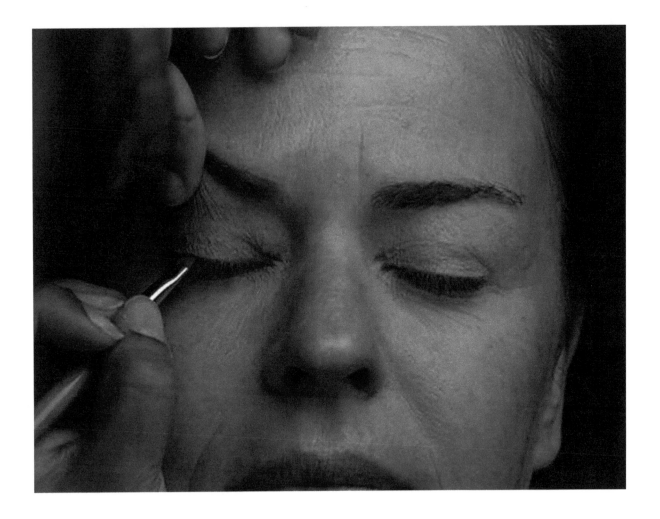

Mascara

Mascara is used to define, thicken and curl eyelashes to frame the eyes, and the options are seemingly endless, but the main types are Volumising, Lengthening and Curling mascaras.

Volumising

These mascaras are suitable for someone with fine or thin eyelashes. They work by building thickness through ingredients such as polymers and waxes, so the formula sticks to the lashes as well as the product itself, creating a fuller look. Volumising wands are usually longer with fine, evenly-spaced bristles to ensure good coverage.

Lengthening

These mascaras are suitable for someone with short lashes and are most effective after using an eyelash curler. They have a thinner formula so that the liquid is easily transferred onto the lash, thus covering each one completely from root to tip. Bristles on lengthening wands are usually shorter and closer together to ensure the mascara glides on the whole lash.

Curling

These mascaras are suitable for someone who doesn't like to use an eyelash curler, but wants to create a wide-eyed look. Like the volumising mascara, the formula is thicker and includes polymers, but the wand will usually be tightly packed and curved to encourage the lashes to curl naturally.

Within each type of mascara, there are two further options: waterproof and non-waterproof.

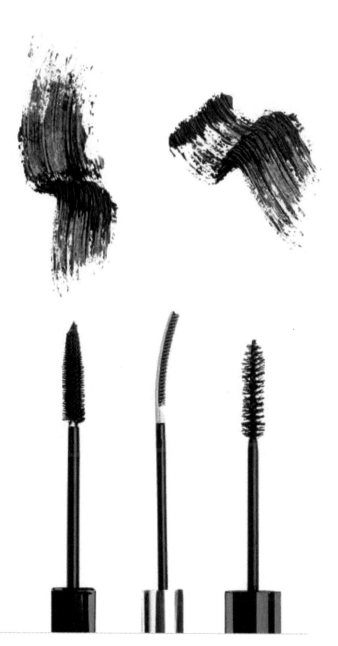

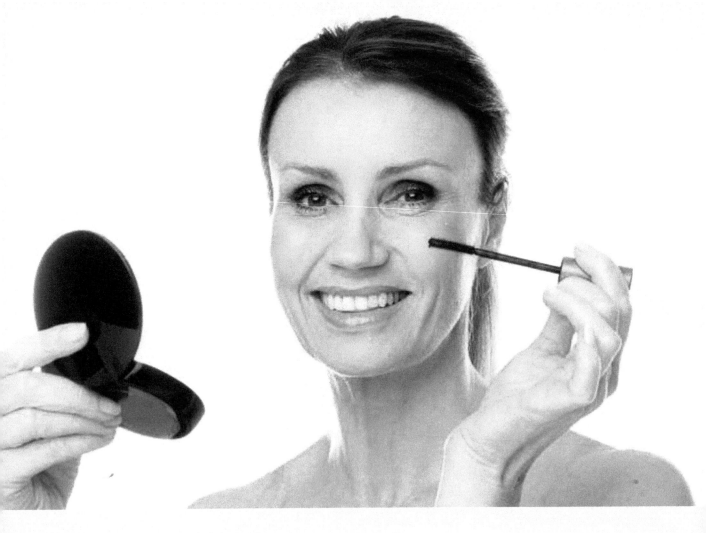

Waterproof Mascara

The benefit of waterproof mascaras is that they last a long time and won't run or smudge when exposed to any form of water, be that rain, the sea, tears or sweat. The downside is that they feel heavier and will only be taken off properly using an oil-based mascara removal solution. Waterproof mascaras are not designed for daily use as they dry out the lashes and removal can be harsh to the whole eye area.

Non-waterproof Mascara

These mascaras smudge and run more easily and are unlikely to last a whole day and night, but they are lighter to wear and easier to clean off before you retire for the evening. It is best to wear non-waterproof mascara on a regular basis and save the waterproof options for special occasions.

Take extra care of mascara products as you can risk transferring bacteria to the eye and getting an infection. If you have used any products while you have had an eye infection, you will need to throw out the items and restock otherwise you will risk a repeat infection.

Blush

Blusher is designed to help contour your face with a little colour and, like foundation, it comes in a variety of forms.

Powder Blush

Applied with a brush, loose powder blush is best for oily skin and can give long-lasting colour which can be built up to be as dense as you wish.

Cream Blush

Cream blush comes in tube or stick form, as well as in small pots or compact cases. While cream can be blended in more easily than powder, it will also give a stronger colour from the start, so apply sparingly and blend with your fingertips. Cream blush will also moisturise your skin and so is suitable for dry or more mature skin.

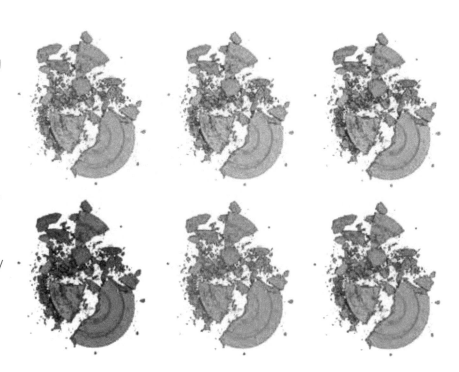

Gel or Liquid Blush

Many liquid blushers are oil-free and therefore are suitable for oily to normal skin. Liquid blushers are thinner in consistency, while gels are not as runny. Typically these are fast-drying blushers and so do not spread or blend as easily, and they are heavily pigmented, so a little goes a long way.

Shimmer or Bronzer

These light powders are great for dusting the whole face, not just the cheeks, and are designed to add warmth and shimmer to your makeup, enhancing naturally tanned skin. They are particularly effective on darker skin to give a healthy glow.

Lipstick

Lipsticks are designed to enhance the colour of your lips and come in a range of finishes, as well as a selection of formats. For any lipstick to take hold however, your lips should be well moisturised. To keep your lips in tip top kissable condition, apply an edible scrub once a week and finish with some soothing balm. Make your own lip scrub by mixing 1 teaspoon of fine brown sugar with 1 teaspoon of organic honey.

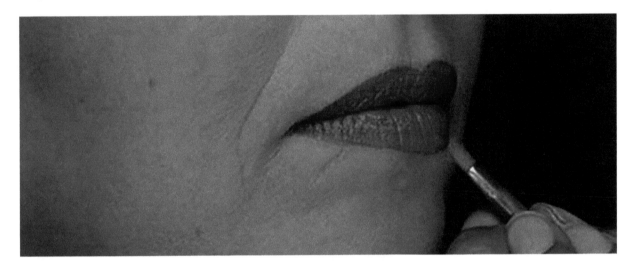

Matte Lipstick

These traditional sticks are great for applying a flat, natural-looking colour and can help your lips appear smoother.

Moisturising Lipstick

If your lips are very dry, even with a regular moisturising scrub and balm, try a moisturising lipstick to nourish your lips while colouring them. Because of the additional moisture, these lipsticks will leave your lips looking shiny.

Satin Lipstick

Satin and sheer lipsticks will also provide additional moisture for dry or chapped lips as they have a high oil content. Beware that the colour on the pack may appear darker than the applied version, and you are likely to need to reapply throughout the day.

Pearl Lipstick

Also known as frosted, these lipsticks will leave your lips with a shimmer so that they sparkle and glisten. As a result of the formula, they can feel very heavy on the lips and leave them dry so are best saved for occasional use.

Long Wearing Lipsticks

Harder working versions of normal lipsticks are available, and while they may mean you don't have to keep reapplying your makeup, they may feel heavier and require additional moisturising before use.

Lip Gloss

This lipstick is liquid rather than solid and makes the lips shine, as well as enhancing the appearance of the shape. A clear gloss can be applied over a traditional matte colour for an extra shine and protection.

Lip Liner

A liner can be used to outline the lips and give increased or decreased definition to the shape and size of the mouth as required. You can either use the same colour as your lipstick, or a shade darker for heightened definition.

You should not reuse lipstick, liner, gloss or balm if you have applied it directly when you were infected with a cold sore. If you used a finger to apply balm once and then washed your hands, the remaining balm should remain uninfected.

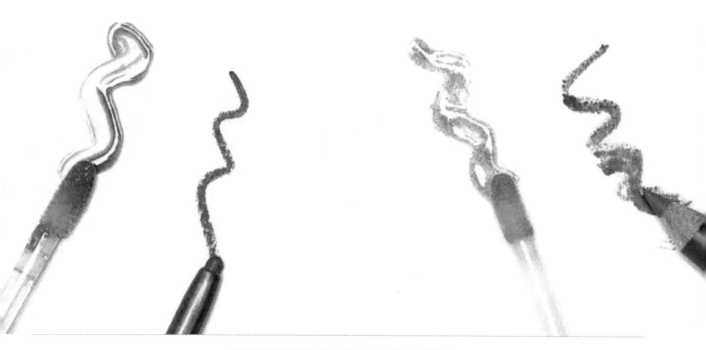

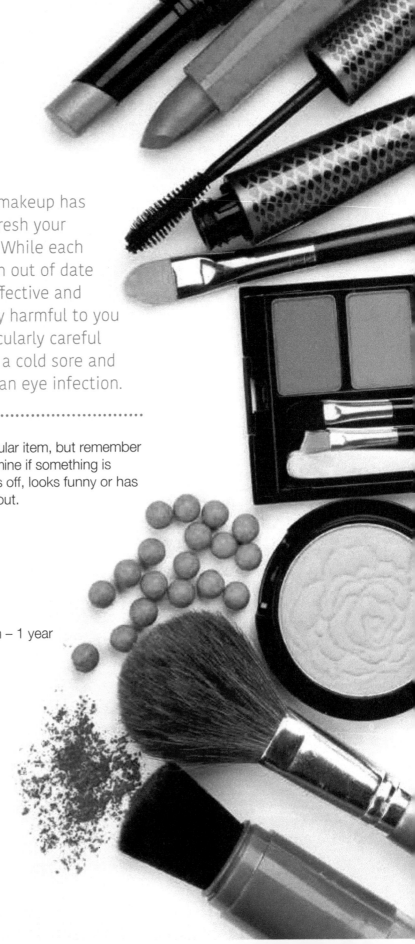

MAKEUP SHELF LIFE

As with all beauty products, makeup has a shelf life so it's best to refresh your products on a regular basis. While each item has its own life span, an out of date product is likely to be less effective and harder to apply, than actually harmful to you however you should be particularly careful with lip products if you have a cold sore and eye makeup if you have had an eye infection.

Here's a guide to the shelf life of regular item, but remember to use your eyes and nose to determine if something is past its best before date – if it smells off, looks funny or has changed consistency, then throw it out.

Powder Foundation – 2 years
Liquid Foundation – 12-18 months
Eye shadow – 3 years
Pencil Eyeliner – 3 years
Liquid Eyeliner – 3-4 months
Mascara – 3-4 months Cream Blush – 1 year
Powder Blush – 2 years
Lipstick – 1-2 years
Lip Liner – up to 3 years

With any liquid products in a tube, don't pump the wand in and out as it exposes the liquid to air and dries it out faster.

MAKEUP INGREDIENTS

As with all beauty products, you should aim for makeup that is as natural as possible, but regardless there are a few nasties that you should look out for and avoid if at all possible:

Parabens

These preservatives have received a lot of media attention in the last decade as they have been linked to an increased risk of breast cancer. The chemicals that prevent the growth of bacteria in your makeup also mimic oestrogen and are absorbed through the skin and many have been linked to breast tumours.

Propylene Glycol

This organic alcohol is often used as a skin-conditioner, but it's also a well-known skin irritant and has been linked to dermatitis and hives.

Bismuth Oxychloride

Often found in mineral powder foundation, this natural ingredient is an irritant to the majority of people, causing itching, redness and inflammation, particularly when the person sweats.

BHA (butylated hydroxyanisole) and BHT (butylated hydroxytoluene)

These synthetic antioxidants act as preservatives, but are also thought to cause cancer, cause allergic reactions and interrupt hormone function.

Mineral Oil

Another preservative, this petroleum by-product clogs the skin's pores and prevents it from eliminating toxins. As it slows down the skin's natural regeneration process, it also results in premature ageing.

Heavy Metals – Lead, Mercury, Cadmium, Arsenic and Nickel among others

Various heavy metals have been found in makeup and those products tend to have two or more of the most worrying metals. These elements build up in the body and cause various health problems over time, including cancer, neurological problems, memory loss, mood swings, kidney and renal problems, headaches, vomiting, nausea and dermatitis.

TIP: You can check your lipstick for the presence of heavy metals by rubbing it on the shiny side of a piece of aluminium foil. Rub the same patch in a circle with a tissue for 10 seconds – if it comes away black, there are heavy metals present in your makeup, if it is clear, then it is ok.

MAKEUP TOOLS

Once you've chosen your makeup you'll need the right tools of the trade, but this doesn't mean going out and spending a small fortune on brushes, sponges and every piece of kit available. Instead, if you carefully select a few good brushes, you can complete your application without too much fuss. In fact, sometimes it's better to invest in a few quality brushes over lots of expensive makeup.

Types of bristles

Good quality makeup brushes consist of densely packed bristles in a shape suitable for its job, and a sturdy wood or plastic handle that feels comfortable to hold. A good brush will cover up the failings of cheaper makeup, whereas a cheap brush will clump even the best makeup.

Natural bristles are best for powders as they are softer and, because they are real, they have a cuticle which helps to hold the pigment. The popular options are sable, squirrel, goat and pony, however many natural bristle companies have been tarnished with animal cruelty and unethical practices.

Synthetic brushes are better for cream or liquid application, and nowadays good quality man-made bristles are almost as good as natural hairs for powders as they have been designed to mimic the cuticle.

Types of brushes

Rather than buy a ready-made kit with 12, 24 or even 32 unnecessary brushes, start with this selection of standard brushes and add any that you find you are really missing – chances are, you won't be!

Foundation brush

A small flat brush used to apply foundation in broad sweeping strokes. A combination of natural and synthetic hairs gives the best of both worlds; a brush that picks up makeup but does not clog. Gone are the days of a foundation sponge, instead choose a brush with a flat shape and a contoured tip to easily blend your makeup.

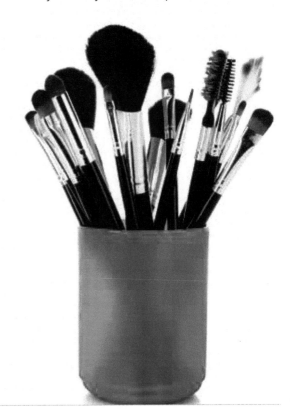

Makeup sponge

Although brushes are generally considered to be the best method to apply foundation, some people still favour makeup sponges.

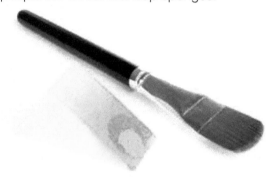

Concealer brush

A small, stiff, flat brush which allows precision blending to cover blemishes. Opt for synthetic bristles to avoid clogging.

Jumbo/Powder brush

A medium-large, round-headed brush for applying powder to specific areas of the face such as forehead, nose and chin which can tend to be greasy.

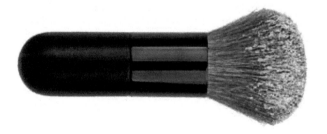

Blush Brush

A slightly smaller, dome-shaped brush for contouring your cheeks with blush, bronzer or highlights. Search for a long-handled brush with a medium-sized head with the silkiest feel you can afford.

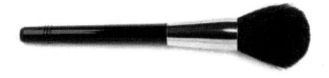

Eye shadow lid brush

A small brush of very densely packed soft bristles which feels smooth and silky to the touch. Choose a half moon shape for precision work in a tight area.

Mascara brush

There are a range of mascara brushes available to help you achieve stunning looking lashes. Whatever the shape of the brush, one with long bristles will help you define your lashes while one with shorter bristles can achieve a thick application.

Rubber bristles tend to give a smooth, even coverage, helping you to build up layers in hard to reach parts, while a curved brush will give your lashes extra curl and lift and work best with smudge-proof mascaras.

Eyelash comb

Run a specialist comb through your lashes after applying mascara to separate and define your lashes from root to tip.

EYEBRUSH GUIDE

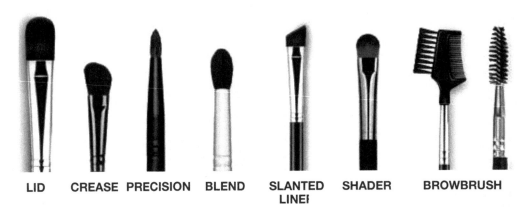

LID   CREASE   PRECISION   BLEND   SLANTED LINEI   SHADER   BROWBRUSH

Lip brush

A small, firm but bendable tip of synthetic bristles for applying lipstick in a controlled way. They often come with a retractable tip to be stored in a handbag without mess.

Eyelash curler

Mascara will help define your eyelashes, but even the best formula has its limits. If you really want your lashes to curl and stand out, try a good quality eyelash curler. Easy and painless to use, this clever gadget will gently curl even the most stubbornly straight lashes and will make them look even longer, allowing your mascara to do its work

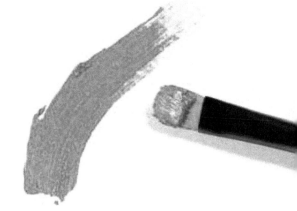

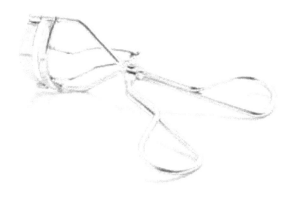

Oil blotting paper

A makeup kit is not complete without oil blotting papers. These little squares can make a big difference when you're out and about – keep them on hand, even in the smallest purse, to blot away any excess oil discreetly and quickly, particularly if someone whips out a camera.

Cotton buds

Likewise, cotton buds can rescue any makeup mistakes such as eye shadow applied too heavily, some eyeliner drawn too far, smudged mascara or a nail polish error. These cheap versatile tools should always be in your makeup bag, travel case and purse to help out whenever you need.

BRUSH CLEANING

With a little care and maintenance, good quality makeup brushes will serve you a long time, which is why it is worth investing in a decent set to start. Some brushes need more regular TLC than others to make sure that you're keeping them in the best possible condition.

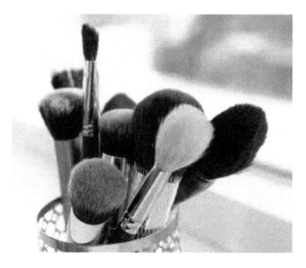

You can buy makeup brush cleaner from the drugstore which can be sprayed on to a tissue to wipe brushes on a daily basis. For a deeper clean, mix a weak solution of mild baby shampoo in some warm water and wash the brushes thoroughly. Once you've washed your brushes, lay them to dry flat on a towel, ideally with the handle slightly raised so that moisture doesn't collect in the casing holding the bristles.

Foundation and concealer brushes

These are the most important brushes to keep clean as they get the most use. Rinse them through after every use to help keep their shape, prevent the makeup clogging or inadvertently spreading oil or dirt from your skin.

Powder brushes

A powder brush won't clog as quickly, so you only need to wash the bristles once a week to keep these tools clean and in perfect condition.

Eye shadow brush

These brushes don't need cleaning as often and can be rinsed out once a month to maintain good condition.

Eyelash curler

Wipe the curlers clean with a makeup wipe once a week and replace the rubber pads regularly to keep your curl perfect.

Blusher brush

Like the eye shadow brush, the blusher brush doesn't need cleaning as often and can be rinsed out once a month to maintain good condition.

Lip brushes

These brushes should also be washed after every use, even if you use the same colour each time, to prevent a build-up of bacteria and the bristles going stiff.

Makeup sponge

If you are using makeup sponges, wash them on a weekly basis in a mild detergent and discard after use for a month.

COLOUR THEORY

Many women don't experiment with makeup because they are unsure what colours to wear, while others just stick with the same two shades they have always worn. Understanding the principles of colour theory will allow you to be confident that you are wearing the best colours to enhance your natural beauty.

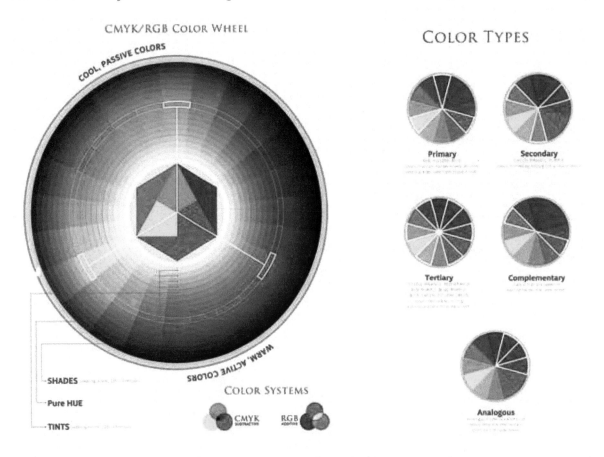

CMYK/RGB COLOR WHEEL

COOL, PASSIVE COLORS

WARM, ACTIVE COLORS

SHADES

Pure HUE

TINTS

COLOR SYSTEMS

CMYK

RGB

COLOR TYPES

Primary

Secondary

Tertiary

Complementary

Analogous

CLASSIC COLOR SCHEMES

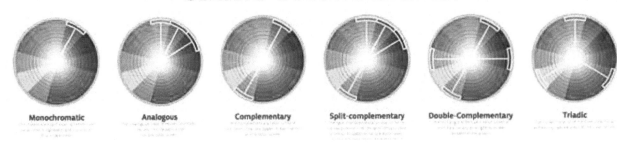

Monochromatic

Analogous

Complementary

Split-complementary

Double-Complementary

Triadic

Before we look at the technical elements, first we need to understand a little more about the formation of colour. If you cast your mind back to art classes in school, you will remember that there are only three primary colours – red, blue and yellow. All other colours are made up from mixing those three: secondary colours are the product of mixing primary colours and are purple, orange and green, while tertiary colours are blends in between primary and secondary colours such as violet and red-orange.

The pure colour is called the hue, but it can be altered in three ways: tint lightens the hue with white, shade darkens the hue with black, while tone changes the hue with grey. Colours with a blue base are known as cool, while yellow based colours are warm, although you can achieve a warm version of a cool colour by adding yellow.

Once you understand the colour wheel, you can easily use it to work out which colours go together. There are four main ways to choose appropriate colour harmonies so that they are pleasing to the eye: monochromatic, analogous, complementary, and triadic.

Monochromatic schemes

This simply focuses on one colour hue, but uses different tones, shades and tints within that restriction to add depth to the look.
It's an easy way of knowing that all elements of makeup will match and is a safe place to start experimenting.

Analogous schemes

These use two or three hues which sit side-by-side on the colour wheel to give one colour scheme with varying shades and hues. The colours blend well and can be used to easily change light daytime makeup to a more dramatic evening look.

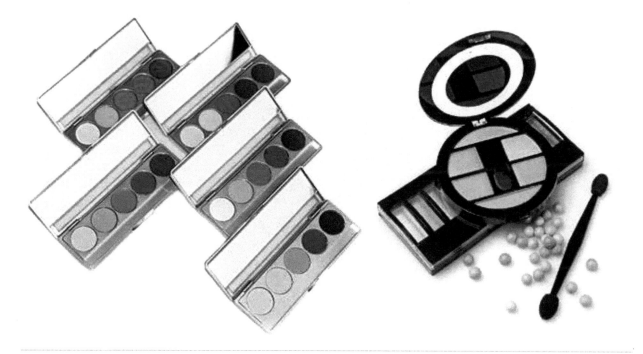

Complementary colour schemes

Using hues on opposite sides of the wheel, complementary colour schemes give a more dramatic look, while the triadic look uses three hues at equidistant points forming a triangle on the colour wheel for a fun, impactful image. (Refer to colour wheel image pg 28)

For example:
VIOLET is opposite to YELLOW on the colour wheel

RED is opposite to GREEN on the colour wheel

BLUE is opposite to ORANGE on the colour wheel.

What does this translate to in the world of eyeshadows?

If your eyes are blue for example look for versions of the colour orange (not PURE ORANGE) such as rusts, copper, coral would be the most effective in making the blue colour in blue eyes stand out.

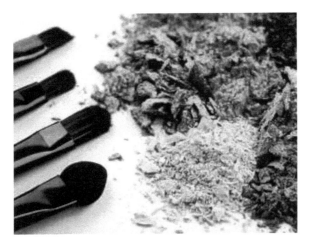

How to make your eye colour stand out

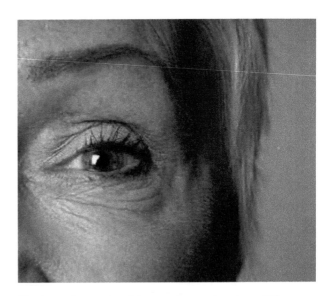

Find a colour wheel (see colour wheel pg 28) and work out where your shade of blue, green, hazel (if your eyes have more of an amber colour to them then they fall into the warmer tone of hazel and if they have more of a green to them then they fall into the cooler tone of hazel) or brown eyes (are they a deep brown almost black brown? (cool) Or are they more of an orange based brown (warm))?

Eye shadow is meant to make your eyes stand out, so complementary colours work best. If you have blue eyes (blue is naturally a cool tone), warm yellow based colours such as terracotta, rusty browns, coppers and bronzes will help your eyes stand out.

If you have green eyes, you should err more towards reds and purples.

While brown eyes can hold their own against most colours.

Eye shadow palettes tend to come in a

range of analogous colours (see analogous colour scheme image above), so once you have chosen your hue you can add depth and highlight with tint, shade and tone. Darker colours can be used for definition, while lighter colours can highlight areas and be used for blending.

Colour Theory applies to eye shadow, blusher and lipstick, and is based on the colour of your eyes, hair and skin tone.

As well as looking at the colour of your eyes and skin tone, you also need to consider your seasonal palette. Look objectively at your image in the mirror and establish where you fall in the following three categories for your primary and secondary characteristics.

The resulting four pure groups are Winter (strong and vivid), Autumn (strong yet muted), Summer (delicate and light) and Spring (delicate and warm), with another four intermediate groups bridging the gaps. Once you have established your colouring, you can begin to see which colours would suit you best, which shades will look ok on you, neither good nor bad, and which ones you should avoid.

DEEP-DARK	LIGHT
Your dark hair and dark eyes are prominent when people see you for the first time.	Your eyes will be light blue or green, but not brown, and your natural hair colour is fair.

SOFT-MUTED	CLEAR
Sometimes called 'mousy', Soft-muted looks are neutral and can lend themselves to being either light or rich.	If your eyes are piercing and your hair is a striking colour, you are Clear if you have a bright crisp look.

WARM	COOL
If you have an all-over glow, with rich earthy tones to your look, your dominant characteristic is Warm.	Ash blonde or grey hair, with grey-blue or soft coloured eyes give an overall Cool look.

COOL SKIN TONES

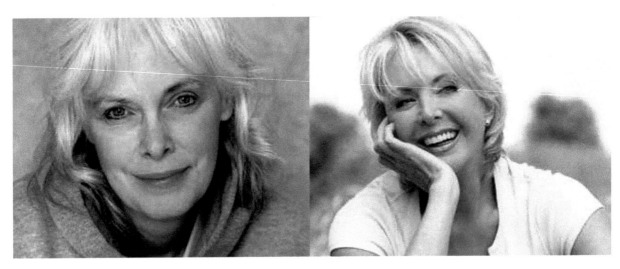

Winter (left) and Summer (Right)

A cool skin tone has more of a blue undertone which is why cooler tones appear to have rosier cheeks. Cooler skin tones also look better wearing silver than gold. As they age their hair goes more of a pure white or silver colour (rather than their warmer toned sisters that go more of a yellow based grey). These women look best when they choose colours from the left hand side of the colour wheel with a blue base to it.

This does not mean that you can only wear purples, blues, or greens. It just means that when you look for colours-any colour at all, it means that red, violet and yellow need to have been mixed from a blue base. If you look at the colour wheel you can wear a more blue based violet (ultramarine violet) instead of a red based violet.

Below is a chart of colours you can use if you have more of a cool tone to your skin. Notice that none of these colours have an orange undertone to them, they're blue or pink based. And this is what you need to look

out for when purchasing lipsticks, eye shadows, foundation and even clothing or accessories that you will wear close to your face. Notice also that there are fewer browns to choose from and that the browns have more of a charcoal base to them and greys also have more of a blue base to them.

Notice that in the **Winter Colour Palette** that the colours are more intense and that with the Summer Colour Palette that the colours are softer. This is because people with a winter palette have more depth of colour to their skin. Winter tones range from the most ivory white in skin to the darkest shade of brown/black.

Summer Skin Tones on the other hand are a little less intense (see the example of the Summer woman above compared to her Winter counterpart) with regards to the amount/depth of colour in the skin. For this reason they suit more watered down or more pastel versions of the same colours

A warm skin toned person has a yellow or

Getting the right tone of colour for your skin will make your skin come to life, your eyes sparkle and your teeth appear brighter.

Getting the colour wrong when you're a cooler tone will make your skin appear sallow

and lifeless, the whites of your eyes will appear more yellow and so will your teeth.

Blue based lip products suit cool coloured skin types. These colours were blended from the left hand side of the colour wheel (see page 28)

Winter Colour Palette:

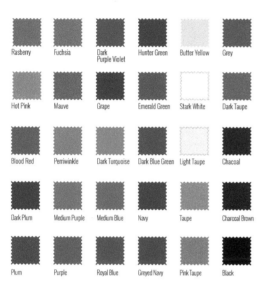

Rasberry	Fuchsia	Dark Purple Violet	Hunter Green	Butter Yellow	Grey
Hot Pink	Mauve	Grape	Emerald Green	Stark White	Dark Taupe
Blood Red	Perriwinkle	Dark Turquoise	Dark Blue Green	Light Taupe	Chacoal
Dark Plum	Medium Purple	Medium Blue	Navy	Taupe	Charcoal Brown
Plum	Purple	Royal Blue	Greyed Navy	Pink Taupe	Black

Summer Colour Palette:

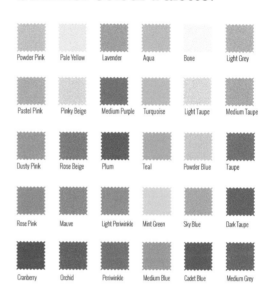

Powder Pink	Pale Yellow	Lavender	Aqua	Bone	Light Grey
Pastel Pink	Pinky Beige	Medium Purple	Turquoise	Light Taupe	Medium Taupe
Dusty Pink	Rose Beige	Plum	Teal	Powder Blue	Taupe
Rose Pink	Mauve	Light Periwinkle	Mint Green	Sky Blue	Dark Taupe
Cranberry	Orchid	Periwinkle	Medium Blue	Cadet Blue	Medium Grey

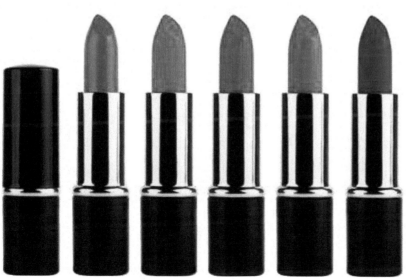

Blue based lip products suit cool coloured skin types. These colours were blended from the left hand side of the colour wheel

WARM SKIN TONES

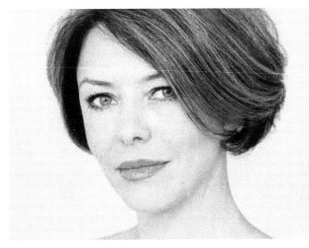 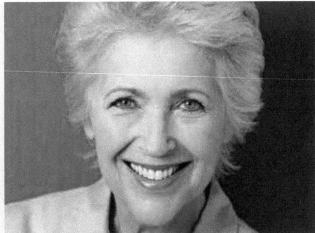

Autumn (left) and Spring (Right)

golden base to the skin, someone who tans easily, with hair that naturally throws off warmer copper tones in the sunlight and who looks good in gold accessories.

Below is a chart of colours you can use if you have more of a warm tone to your skin. Notice there are greens and blues on the chart which are found on the left hand side of the colour wheel (normally associated with cool tones)-however, none of these colours have a blue undertone to them, they're more orange/red based.

You'll also notice that there are a lot more browns available for warmer toned women to wear however the browns are more of a yellow, orange or red based brown. Greys tend to be more of a yellow based grey. And white is more of an ivory white (otherwise known as off-white, with a yellow base to it.

Remember this when purchasing lipsticks, eye shadows, foundation and even clothing or accessories that you will wear close to your face.

Notice that in the **Autumn Colour Palette** that the colours are more intense and that with the Spring Colour Palette that the colours are softer. This is because people with an autumn palette have more depth of colour to their skin.

Autumn Colour Palette:

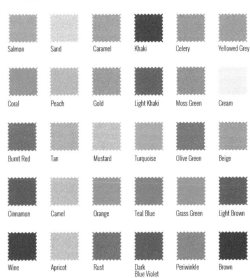

Salmon	Sand	Caramel	Khaki	Celery	Yellowed Grey
Coral	Peach	Gold	Light Khaki	Moss Green	Cream
Burnt Red	Tan	Mustard	Turquoise	Olive Green	Beige
Cinnamon	Camel	Orange	Teal Blue	Grass Green	Light Brown
Wine	Apricot	Rust	Dark Blue Violet	Periwinkle	Brown

Spring Skin Tones on the other hand are a little less intense (see the example of the Spring women above compared to their Autumn counterpart) with regards to the amount/depth of colour in the skin. For this reason they suit more watered down or more pastel versions of the same colours

Spring Colour Palette:

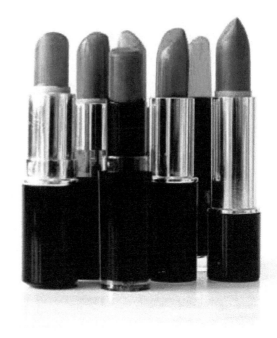

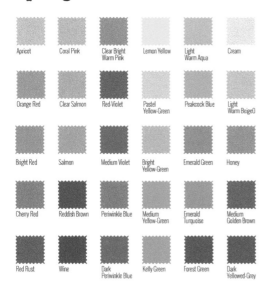

Apricot	Coral Pink	Clear Bright Warm Pink	Lemon Yellow	Light Warm Aqua	Cream
Orange Red	Clear Salmon	Red-Violet	Pastel Yellow-Green	Peakcock Blue	Light Warm Beige0
Bright Red	Salmon	Medium Violet	Bright Yellow-Green	Emerald Green	Honey
Cherry Red	Reddish Brown	Periwinkle Blue	Medium Yellow-Green	Emerald Turquoise	Medium Golden Brown
Red Rust	Wine	Dark Periwinkle Blue	Kelly Green	Forest Green	Dark Yellowed-Grey

Getting the right tone of colour for your skin will make your skin glow, your eyes sparkle and your teeth appear brighter.

Getting the colour wrong when you're a warmer tone will wash you out and overwhelm your natural colouring.

These reds/oranges suit warmer toned skins. Notice that the reds, pinks and browns have more of an orange/yellow base to them.

When choosing a blush, the colour should not be darker than your natural flush if you were to run once around the block. If you have a cool skin tone, the lighter, ashier blushes will work better, whereas warm skin tones can wear stronger, darker pinks with a warm shimmer.

Lipstick should not only work with your eye shadow and blush colours, but also help make the most of the size of your lips. If your lips are thin, use a lighter shade to make them appear fuller, while full lips can be tamed with a darker shade to make them smaller. A dark shade lipstick against a cool skin tone will slightly age the wearer, while a warm bright colour against a warm skin tone will keep the wearer looking young.

Finally, you might like to choose your colours to reflect your personality or provoke certain reactions in others. Here are the most common meanings and psychological reactions to colours:

Red:
Passion, Love, Anger, Power, Sexy

Orange:
Energy, Happiness, Vitality, Halloween

Yellow:
Happiness, Hope, Bright, Summer

Green:
New Beginnings, Abundance, Nature, Growing

Blue:
Calm, Responsible, Sadness/Depression, Winter

Pink:
Sweet, Lovely, First Love, Flowers

Purple:
Creativity, Royalty, Wealth, Romance

Black:
Mystery, Elegance, Evil

Grey:
Moody, Conservative, Formality, Dull

White:
Purity, Cleanliness, Virtue, Light, Snow

Brown:
Nature, Wholesomeness, Dependability, Autumn

Tan or Beige:
Conservative, Piety, Dull

Cream or Ivory:
Calm, Elegant, Purity

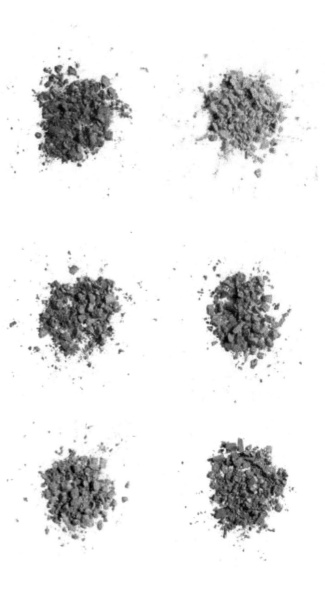

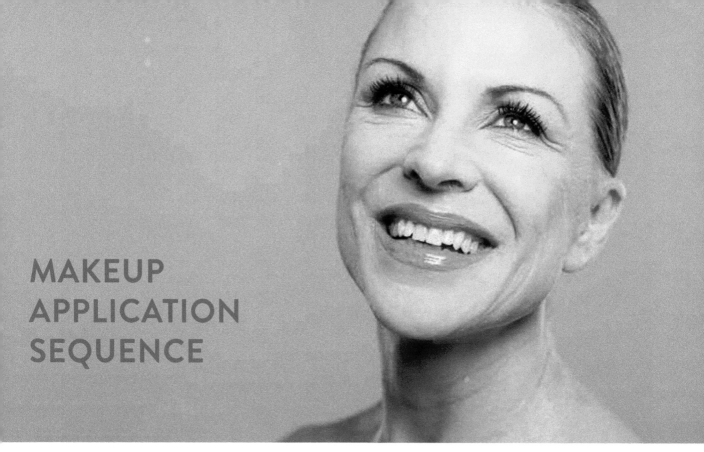

MAKEUP APPLICATION SEQUENCE

Makeup works best when it highlights your natural beauty. This is why it is so important to understand the colour theory, your skin tone, hair and eye colouring, as well as what suits you best. While you can use makeup to create a statement image, it is most effective when used to brighten your own features, enhance your true looks and help you look your best.

An unflattering makeup application will have the same impact as a dramatic look and draw attention to you, whereas a carefully blended application which augments your own beauty will give you confidence and make you seem more appealing.

Although foundation sounds like it should be the starting point, it is best to apply eye makeup prior to foundation as it is a lot easier to wipe off any spilt coloured eye shadow from clean skin, rather than removing and redoing foundation. There is nothing worse than perfectly applying your foundation only to have to start again because you've had fall out from eye shadow.

However, you can complete the base of the eyes after foundation and concealer as it gives the base section of your eye makeup longer wear, while creating a barrier to stop your eye makeup running down your face. Apply your darker contour colour to the outer edge of your lower lash line and blend inwards finishing just before the tear duct. Make sure the majority of your eye shadow pigment is on the outer section of the lower lash line and that only a small amount is blended inwards or the look can be too heavy.

Finish with some blush, lipstick and mascara, and you are ready to let your beauty radiate for the day.

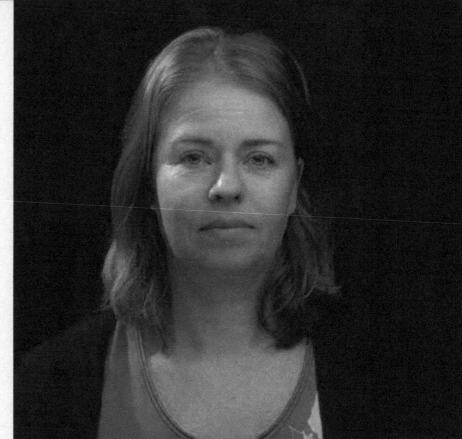

Makeover
before

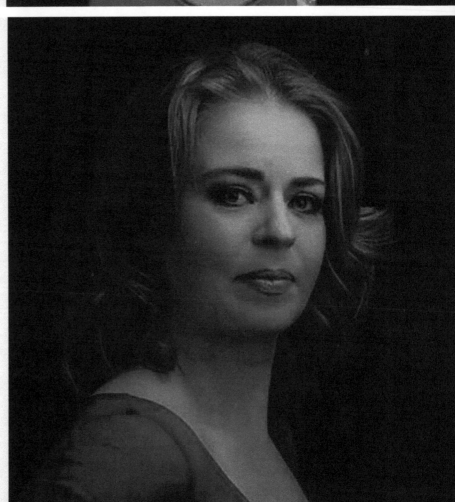

Makeover
after

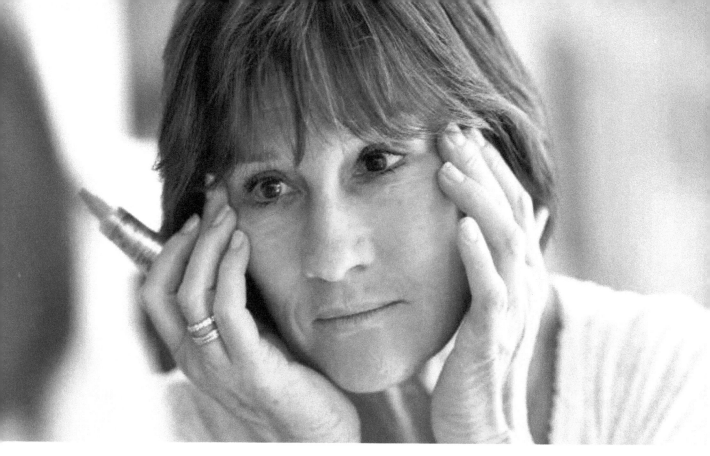

Applying Concealer

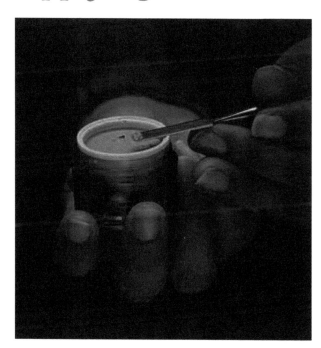

To conceal your under-eye area, find your orbital bone by pressing around the eye area. If you press around your lower lash area you'll feel a semicircular hollow. This is the outer limit as well as the starting point for your concealer application. Simply apply your concealer along this bone and into the hollow around the tear ducts, and then blend your concealer upwards and outwards towards the lower lash line.
(as indicated by the red arrow)

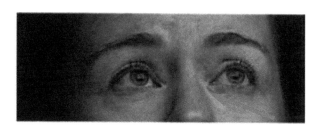

It is important not to apply your concealer from the lower lash line downwards, but to blend upwards otherwise it will look cakey and inadvertently highlight any wrinkles. If you feel that your concealer is caking and is really not sitting well on the lines around your eyes, simply wet your sponge so that it is moist and blend the concealer out.

As the skin matures any sun damage picked up over the years becomes more prominent, with blemishes such as age spots and pigmentation (brown discolourations on the skin), capillary damage (redness around the sides of nose, cheeks and sometimes chin), moles and skin cancers starting to appear. This creates a very uneven skin tone, which can easily add an extra 10 years to the appearance of the skin.

This can just as easily be covered and evened out with concealer. As it is slightly thicker in texture than foundation, concealer gives better coverage for any imperfections.

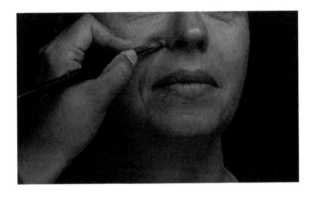

Capillary damage often occurs around the sides of the nose, sometimes extending onto the cheeks, and across the chin. Just dab some concealer onto these unsightly red marks and simply blend either using your fingers or a sponge.

Age spots, also known as sunspots or liver spots, can also be covered in the same way – just remember to keep the concealer within the borders of the pigmentation.

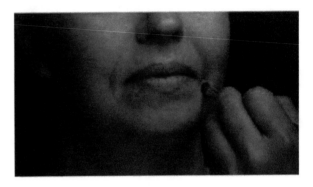

The nasolabial lines that run from the sides of the nose to the outer edges of the mouth, and sometimes extend down from the bottom corners of the lips down the chin, can often have darker areas, particularly at the side of the mouth.

If this is prominent and something that bothers you, then apply concealer to the discoloured skin using a shade lighter than your natural skin tone. This will help brighten the area and visually bring the line forward as it's the darkness of the line that makes it stand out and appear stronger.

Applying a thin amount of concealer around the border of the lip line (particularly to the cupids bow and the lower lip line) will help the problem of lipstick feathering out into the creases around your mouth.

As with other areas, once applied simply blend with either a sponge or your fingers.

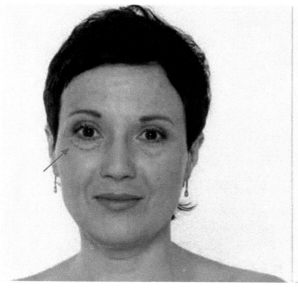
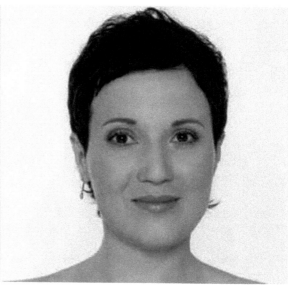

Troubleshooting tips for concealing puffy eyes:

If you suffer from dark puffy circles under eyes, help is at hand with a little concealer carefully applied. Rather than applying your concealer onto the orbital bone and blending up, as shown in the earlier section, the best way to reduce the appearance of eye bags is to dab concealer along the dark line at the base of the puffy bag and blend down onto the cheek bone. The reason for this is that by lightening that section it makes the crease of the bag less obvious and helps blend it into the cheek. It won't get rid of the bag entirely, but it will lessen the puffy appearance.

Alternately, you can start to use specialist eye creams in order to more effectively eliminate dark circles and eye bags. Because the skin under the eye is the thinnest and most delicate, it benefits greatly from extra nourishment and hydration, and many of the products on the market include ingredients that plump and tighten loose skin.

Retinol is perhaps the most common active ingredient in eye creams. A derivative of vitamin A, it helps the skin restore collagen to actively reduce the crevices that cause lines and wrinkles, as well as smoothing out the skin by reducing pore size. Caffeine is often also used to help constrict the blood vessels under the eye to reduce puffiness. A cream containing hyaluronic acid will provide the delicate skin with ultra-hydration and help smooth out the under-eye area. Natural botanics used include horse chestnut, Quercetin and oak. Any product that is applied using a metal roller ball will stimulate the skin with a mini massage and many women keep their eye products in the fridge to improve the soothing quality on tired eyes.

While all these products are pretty amazing, be aware that some can leave a slight film on the skin which means that makeup doesn't adhere so well. Either expect to pay a higher price for one which absorbs well or apply the cream overnight and clean the skin before putting on makeup, otherwise you will need to be careful about blending concealer into the eye cream.

Applying Eye Shadow

As we mature, the tissue below the brow bone begins to sag making the eyes appear heavier and often giving the impression of a tired look. Because of this natural change, you will need to adapt the way you apply makeup as wearing eye shadow the same way you did in your twenties can often enhance the lines and heavier lids that you are trying to disguise.

The aim of this section on eye shadow application therefore is to teach you how to apply eye shadow in a way that helps to lift your eyes, making them appear brighter, larger and more open.

- Silky matte eye shadows are best for mature eyes as they blend well into the skin and add natural definition to eyes.

- Stay away from shimmers or glittery eye shadows as they have light reflectors in the colour, which means that it sits on top of the skin and emphasizes the creases and wrinkles around the eyes.

- Simply choosing matte eye shadows instead of shimmer varieties you are able to reduce the appearance of wrinkles and puffiness around the eyes.

Once your concealer has set in, you can begin to apply your eye shadow.

Step 1: Prime the eyelid

By using an eyelid primer, you are providing a smooth even canvas which will improve the eye shadow's ability to adhere to your skin, giving you a stronger eye shadow colour which lasts longer. Invest in a decent eyelid primer. One that is silicon based, rather than oily, is preferable as the latter will break down the foundation, whereas a silicon based eye primer will create a more even base for makeup application. Apply primer all over the eye area.

Step 2: Apply a light eye shadow to your eyelid

Apply a light or skin-coloured eye shadow to the entire top eyelid using an eye shadow brush; a small round head is best. You can either place the shadow to the lid as a wash by simply dragging the brush across the lid, or you can place the lid colour at the base of the top lash line and press or pat the colour all over the lid for a greater intensity of colour on the eyelid.

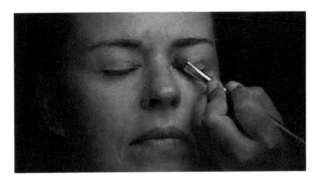

Please note: Only apply the light colour to the eyelid, not the eye socket. If you take the light colour above the natural lid crease or socket line (the join where your lids open) you will emphasize any sagging of the eyes or wrinkles that are present, see the illustration below:

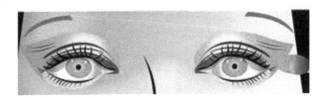

As you can see, when the light colour is brought up and over the natural lid crease line it enhances wrinkles and gives the eyes a tired sagging look – not what we are trying to achieve!

Step 3: Apply a darker contour colour

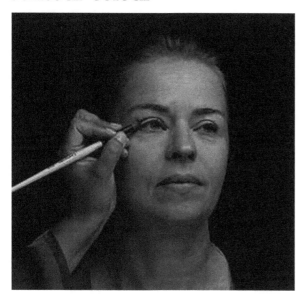

Apply the darker contour colour in a "C" or side-on "V" shape. This darker colour will soon be blended to soften the edges, but it helps reframe your eyes so that they will appear larger and more open.

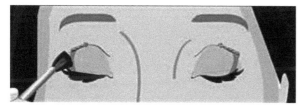

Once the darker contour colour is applied to outer edge of the eyelid, blend upwards and slightly higher than the natural lid crease. This creates the illusion of a larger eye socket and longer eyelids, which ultimately makes your eyes look larger.

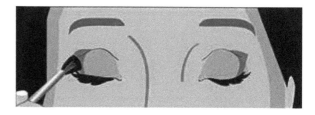

With a blender brush, blend your darker contour colour upwards and outwards.
When blending your eye shadow, ensure that you are using a soft bristled blender brush in either small circular motions or a light feathery backwards and forwards motion for best effect, see illustrations below.

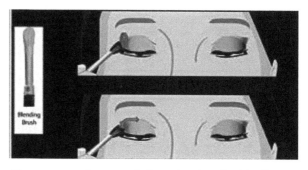

You can apply your darker shadow just to the outer edges like the image above or you can bring the contour all the way to the inner corner of the lid crease. The end result is a matter of personal preference, but the key is to blend upwards and outwards, aiming to soften the edges of your contour line.

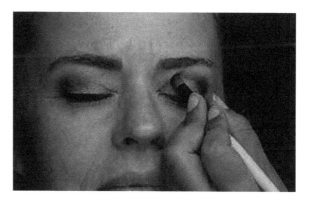

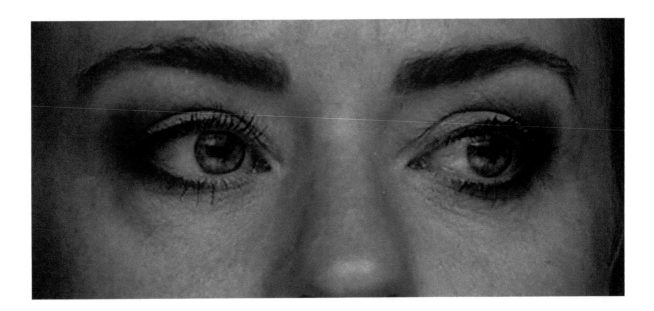

Step 4: Apply a highlight colour

To finish off the eye shadow application, apply a highlight colour just below the brow bone and blend. Placing a lighter colour within your chosen colour range just under the brow bone will help visually lift the eyes and make them look wider still.

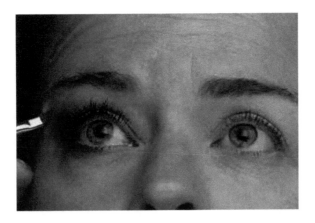

TIP: unless your eyelids are protruding or push outwards it is important to apply a light,

not dark, colour to the lid otherwise your eyes will look as though they have been pushed backwards into the eye socket as per the example below:

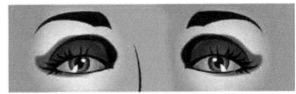

By applying a darker contour colour only slightly above the lid crease line, with a lighter colour over the eyelid will make the eyes appear more open, as per the image below:

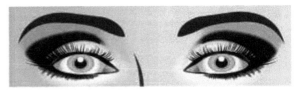

As you can see, the eyeshadow is light on the lid, with a darker colour blended just above the lid crease line and a lighter colour on the brow bone to make the eyes appear more open.

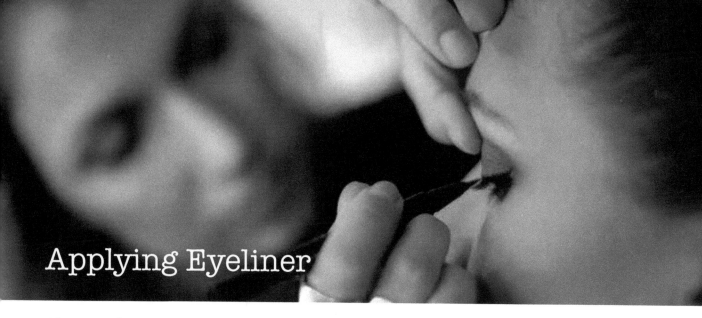

Applying Eyeliner

After you have put on your eye shadow, apply liner to top lash line with your chosen pencil. Ensure the liner is applied as close to the lash line as possible –

If you inadvertently leave a gap between your lashes and your liner, fill it in to make a thicker line rather than leaving it which looks odd. To make your eyes appear even wider, graduate the thickness of your liner by making it thinner at the inside corner and thicker at the outer corner of your eye.

TIP: Hold your skin taught with your fingers while applying your liner to stop any gaps occurring if there are wrinkles on the eyelid.

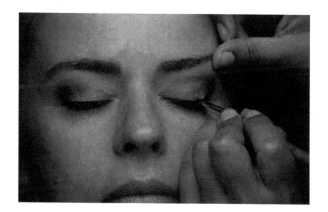

Also, look down but don't close your eyes when you apply your liner as this stretches the skin on the eyelid better than on fully closed eyes.

If you make a mistake while applying eyeliner, or a gap shows up, simply use your angled eyeliner brush or cotton tip to blend the line and give a softer finish.

The same form of eyeliner application is true whether you use a pencil, liquid, gel or eye shadow as liner, but the effects will be different. Liquid and gel liners will give a longer lasting but harder edge, while a pencil and eye shadow will produce a more temporary, softer image.

You can use a gel liner with an angled or slanted eyeliner brush for a longer lasting definition and the advantage of a gel liner is that it is easier to clean it up if you make a mistake.

A liquid liner, for instance, is generally less forgiving and not as easy to work with unless you have had a lot of practise. An advantage of using a liquid liner is that it is the least likely option to smudge once it is dry, so it is great for a full day or a night out socialising.

To achieve the best results with a

SLANDTED
LINER

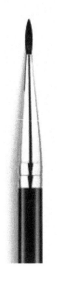

EYELINER
BRUSH
*The pointed tip
will give you a very
precise lash line*

liquid liner, use a brush which has a defined tip like the one below, as it gives a precise application. Begin with a thin line and build up the thickness to the desired width as it is easier to add extra liquid liner than it is to remove it.

If you prefer to use eye shadow as an eyeliner, you can use an angled eye brush and then smudge it with your blender brush. This gives a much softer look than the gel, liquid or pencil liners but still defines the eye perimeter.

TIP: Try all four options when you have the time to see which medium you prefer to use and which look you think best suits each occasion.

Lower Lash Line

Using the same colour as the contour colours used in your eye shadow application, apply a thin line under your lower lashes.

If you feel that your eyes are small and you want them to appear larger you would be

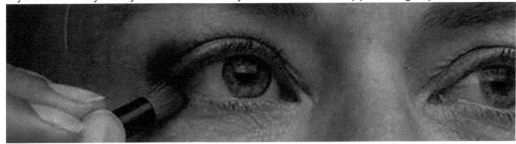

best off only taking the darker contour colour to the outer third of your lower lash line, then using a lighter colour further in to your inner eyes.

If not... feel free to bring the darker contour colour right through to the inner eyes.

TIP: If you have finished applying your eye makeup and think the look is too heavy,

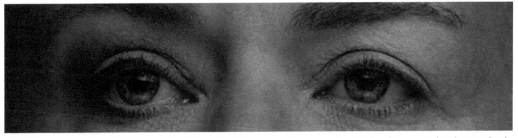

don't overreact and remove it all to start from scratch, try just thinning out the lower lash eyeliner. It's best to practice and make mistakes in your own time so that you get a feel for what you like and can replicate it easily when it matters for a special occasion.

A good quality mascara, whether it's waterproof or not, should be liquid enough to

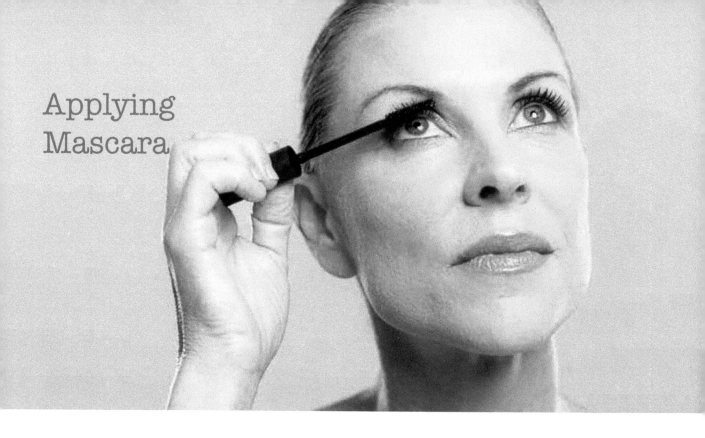

Applying Mascara

The aim of using mascara is to add length and volume to your lashes to frame your eyes and make them appear more youthful and open. Curling your lashes will have a big impact on how enticing your eyes look. This can either be done before applying mascara with a manual lash curler – position as close to the lash line and press to get a natural "J" curl – or after you've coloured your lashes, using a heated curling wand.

apply easily, yet one that dries quickly without flaking. Remember that mascara has a short shelf life, so check the consistency each time you use it to make sure it's still good.

It is important to choose the right mascara brush for the job: a thin mascara brush is great for lengthening the lashes by defining each one from root to tip, thick bristles help to add volume to the lashes and a curved brush helps to shape the lashes to give an eye-opening curl.

Step 1: Preparing the mas-cara

Remove excess mascara formula by wiping the brush along the bottle opening or dabbing on a tissue. Do not pump the wand in and out of the bottle to get rid of any clumps as this will push air into the container and spoil your mascara quicker.

Step 2: Top lashes

Hold the mascara wand horizontally and start with the underside of the top set of lashes. Begin as close to the base as possible and zig zag your brush up the lash. This will help deposit the mascara either side of the lashes thereby giving the lash a thicker appearance. Then drag the wand all the way up the lash and off the tip of the lash to add volume.

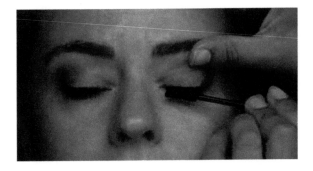

Step 3: Cover all lashes

Adjust the wand left to right and repeat as necessary to ensure full coverage of all lashes.

Step 4: Comb the lashes

Brush the lashes with a clean wand or lash comb to even out application and remove any clumps and allow to dry before applying mascara to the bottom lashes.

Step 5: Bottom lashes

Hold the wand vertically for the bottom set of lashes and slowly move back and forth for a controlled application. Allow lashes to dry, comb through and remove any flakes with a sweep of a powder brush.

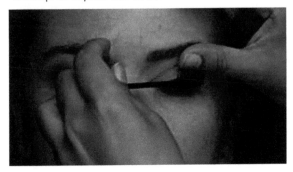

TIP: As you start aging your lashes and brows will become sparser, so adding extra volume and length will help to open up your eyes and give a more youthful appearance. If added length is your main objective, hold your wand vertically and drag the tip of the brush from the base of the lash though to the tip.

Alternately, if you have particularly fine or short lashes, you can use a two-step type of mascara which mimics natural eyelash extensions. A white liquid is added to your lashes first to add length, but it needs to set before using your normal mascara, so apply the base coat to your lashes in the same way as normal mascara and leave to dry for a minute.

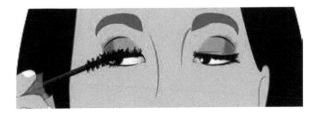

Then apply your normal mascara over the top.

If you have sensitive eyes or find that mascara irritates you, lash tinting might be a better option. A colour with a low level of peroxide (3%) is added to the lashes – usually a blue black (jet black), black or brown – to give definition for around 3-4 weeks. By tinting your lashes once a month, you don't have to worry about applying mascara every day. Speak to your aesthetician if this is something that appeals to you.

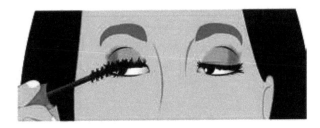

Applying
False Eyelashes

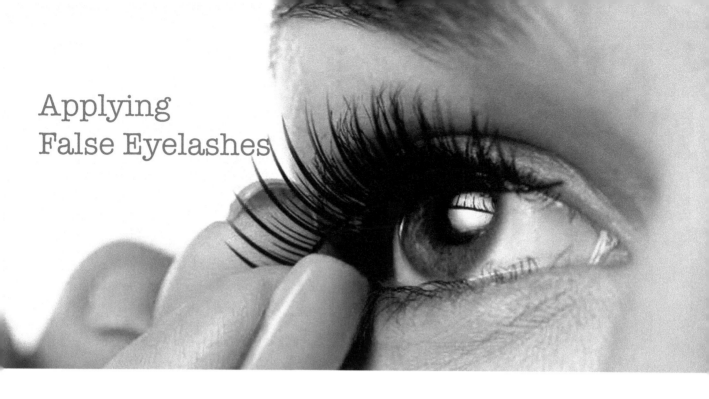

Another way to get killer lashes is to apply a false strip to the top lash line.

Step 1: Prepare the false lashes

Using a small to medium length lash kit, measure and cut each strip to the length of your eyelid. Leaving them too long will drag your eye down and defeat the objective of opening up your eyes.

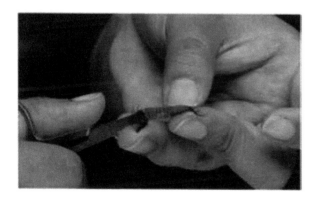

Step 2: Apply the glue

Apply dots of the lash glue along your natural lash line and on the back of the lash strip. Wait 30 seconds until the glue is tacky.

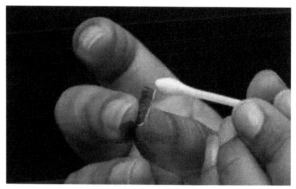

Step 3: Apply the lashes

Hold the false lashes in the middle with a pair of tweezers and carefully place along your lash line. Push the inner side of the strip in first, then gently pat the outer side in place.

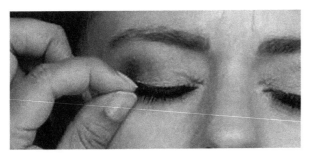

Step 4: Bond to real lashes

You can use the tweezers to pinch the false lashes to your own real lashes for a seamless effect. As soon as they are in place, leave them alone – the more you fiddle with them, the more likely they are to come unstuck.

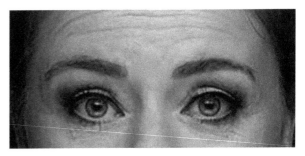

Step 5: Apply makeup

Wait a minute or two for the lashes to fully stick, then add eyeliner and eye shadow in the normal way. Apply mascara to your real lashes only for a fuller effect and to help join them to your strip lash to look more natural.

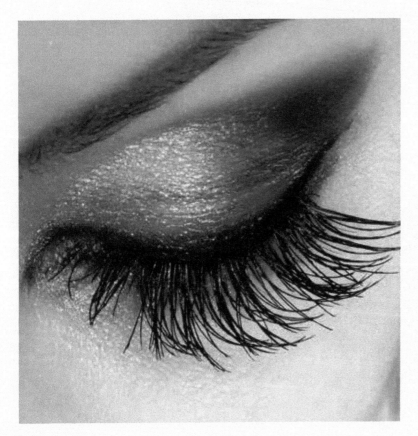

Eyelash Extensions

If you don't want the hassle of fake lashes, you can opt for eyelash extensions. In the same way as hair extensions mini individual silk fibres, which look just like lashes, are attached to your natural lashes.

The lashes will fall out with your natural lashes, so this semi-permanent option can last anywhere between 2-6 weeks before a top up is required. Below is an image of how natural well-applied eyelash extensions can look.

Eyebrows

Eyebrows tend to become either sparse or wiry as you age, but either way they will start requiring more of your attention. When styling the eyebrows, it is important to understand how they should look to maximize your appearance.

Eyebrow Size

The drawing below shows the optimum size of the eyebrow on the left eye. The eyebrow should start at the point directly above the line running from the nostril to the inner corner of the eye. Any hairs that appear beyond that point, towards the other eye, should be removed, either by plucking with tweezers, threading, waxing or by depilatory cream. Never use a razor on your eyebrows as it will stimulate stubbly regrowth.

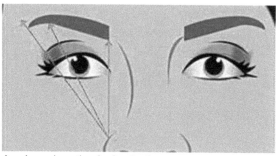

Again using the indent of your nose as your starting point, draw an imaginary line at 45 degrees through the eye, between the pupil and iris. This will give you a reference as to where you should start the arch of your eyebrow.

The last guideline runs from the nostril in a straight line past the outer edge of your lower lash line's end point and onwards to the end of the brow bone. This should be the end of your eyebrows and any hair that lies past that point should be removed as above.

The guidelines on the right eye above helps

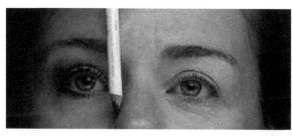

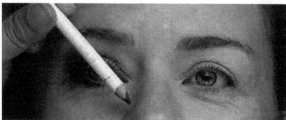

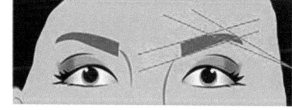

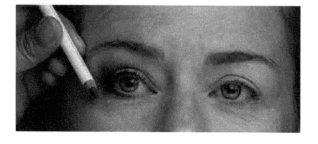

explain the area where it is ok to remove excess hair without taking away too much thickness from your brow. Starting from the base of the brow, create a parallel line at the thickness you want to give you the width of the upward slant. Using the previous diagram to establish the point of the arch, taper the eyebrow down so that it ends at the edge of your eye. Any stray hairs outside these guidelines can be safely removed.

Eyebrow Control

If you find that your eyebrows are wiry and hard to tame, a pair of eyebrow scissors and an eyebrow brush (similar in appearance to a mascara wand) are great tools for getting them under control. Simply comb the eyebrows upward and then trim long and unruly hairs above the natural top line of the brow.

Eyebrow Fill

If you find that your eyebrows have thinned over time as a result of over-plucking, shaving the brows or general hair loss, then there are a few ways to restore the shape of your eyebrows:

1. You can pencil them in

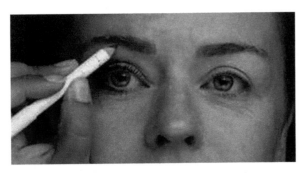

Use short feathery strokes when filling in your missing eyebrows and imagine you are adding in individual hairs, one by one, rather than drawing a straight line which can look quite severe if applied too heavily. Chose a colour that is no more than two shades darker than your natural hair colour. If you had blonde eyebrows then a mousy brown shade is probably the darkest colour you should try.

2. You can powder them in

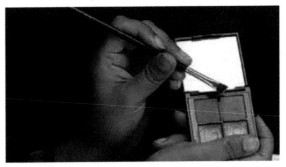

Using the slanted liner, or angled eyebrow brush, you can add colour to your brows using feathery strokes. Aim to follow the natural shape of your brows and fill in any gaps that may exist. As with the pencil, choose a colour within two shades of your natural hair colour.

3. You can apply a gel coat

You can add colour and thicken the appearance of your thinning brows by applying a coloured gel with a brow brush. As with the pencil, choose a colour within two shades of your natural hair colour.

4. You can tint them

You can have your eyebrows tinted to give a semi-permanent colour either at home or professionally by an aesthetician. Avoid black tint as it has an ageing effect and can look quite harsh – a deep brown or charcoal tint will suffice if you have a winter palette. Like eyelash tints, this option will need redoing as your eyebrows naturally grow out.

5. You can tattoo them

Block tattoos can look quite harsh, so it's best to get your brows tattooed with individual strokes which look more natural. While this is the only permanent option to restoring your eyebrows, it's is not for everyone as tattooing can be painful.

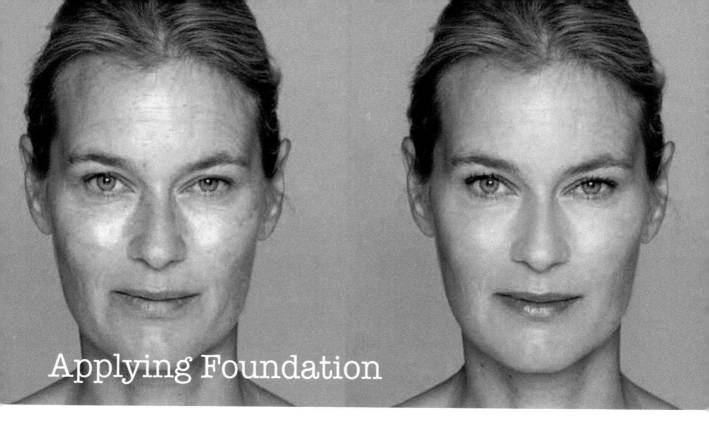

Applying Foundation

Foundation makes the skin look even and smooth when applied well, so take the time to learn how to put on your best face.

Colour

Getting the right colour is crucial as there is nothing worse than seeing a line where the foundation ends, so make sure your foundation matches your neck. The best way to get the right colour is to patch test a few shades on your jaw line – the one that looks like it's disappeared into the skin is the right choice.

Application

Less is more with foundation application on mature skin as it can inadvertently highlight creases and wrinkles if applied too thickly. The concealer provides medium to heavy coverage and will have done the majority of the work in evening out the skin tone. Foundation gives a light to medium coverage to smooth the overall skin.

Tools

What you'll need to create a flawless foundation finish:

1. Sponge or small brush for blending

2. Foundation or kabuki brush

3. Fingertips when you don't have either of the above

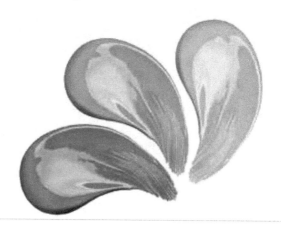

Liquid foundation

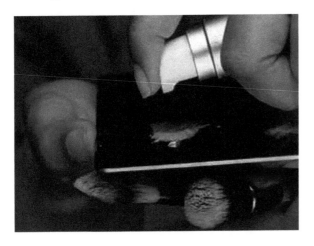

STEP 1: start by applying dots of liquid foundation to the centre of your face, cheeks and forehead.

STEP 2: using either your sponge, foundation brush or fingertips, spread the foundation over the rest of your skin in a stippling motion. Think about pressing the foundation into your skin rather than wiping it across your face. This ensures that your foundation sits flawlessly, giving the skin a buffed look.

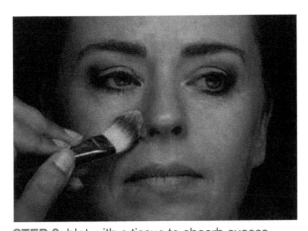

STEP 3: blot with a tissue to absorb excess oils and seal with a light dusting of translucent powder to help the staying power of your foundation.

Powder Foundation

This method can be used either when using a powder foundation or to set liquid foundation with a translucent powder.

STEP 1: a kabuki brush is ideal for applying mineral powder makeup as it holds a lot of powder in the hair of its large head. Simply swirl the brush around your makeup pot and tap off any excess. Apply either in a circular motion all over the face or brush liberally over each section.

STEP 2: however you apply the powder, always finish by brushing in a downwards action so that your facial hairs lie flat.

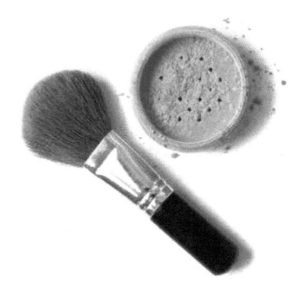

TIP: If setting the liquid foundation with a powder, sometimes the powder might fall into lines and make the skin appear more creased. The best way to overcome this is to apply the powder with a fan brush over areas where more lines appear, such as crow's feet above the cheeks or laughter lines around the mouth. The fan brush gives a light dusting of powder to the face and makes it easier to control the amount of colour that goes onto the skin, whereas larger brushes deposit more powder onto the skin.

Applying Contour

You can contour the face using a liquid foundation, loose powder or even a bronzer. It helps add dimension to your features and can be used to reshape your face if desired.

Colour and Tools

A contour colour – usually one or two shades darker than your natural skin tone – can be applied over your foundation and blended well. A contour brush is shaped with a diagonal end and is designed to give you more control, but you could also use a blush brush flattened between your fingers.

Application

STEP 1: starting under the cheek bone, use the centre of your pupil as your guide – you don't need to bring your contour colour any further in towards the nose than the line of your pupil. Sweep the colour outwards towards your ear, under the jawline and up to the temple.

STEP 2: using a kabuki or blender brush, blend the contour colour into the foundation so that there are no harsh edges. As with foundation, less is definitely more, so start off with a small amount and add more if needed. It's easy to add more, but very difficult to take away when you have too much colour.

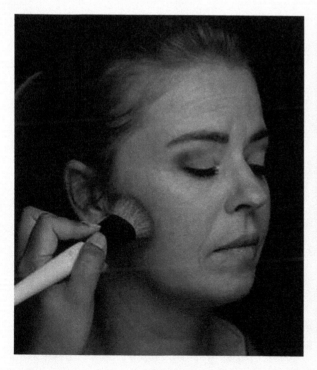 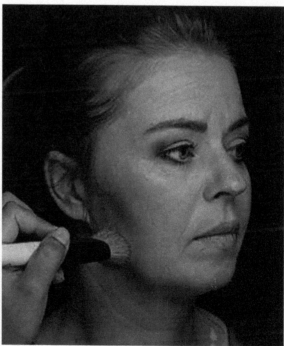

If you want your cheeks to stand out more, then you would contour just underneath the cheek bone to make them appear more uplifted. You can apply contour colour to the temple to define the face, or the jawline if you want to reduce the appearance of jowls, and it can be applied in a large backward "3" shape.

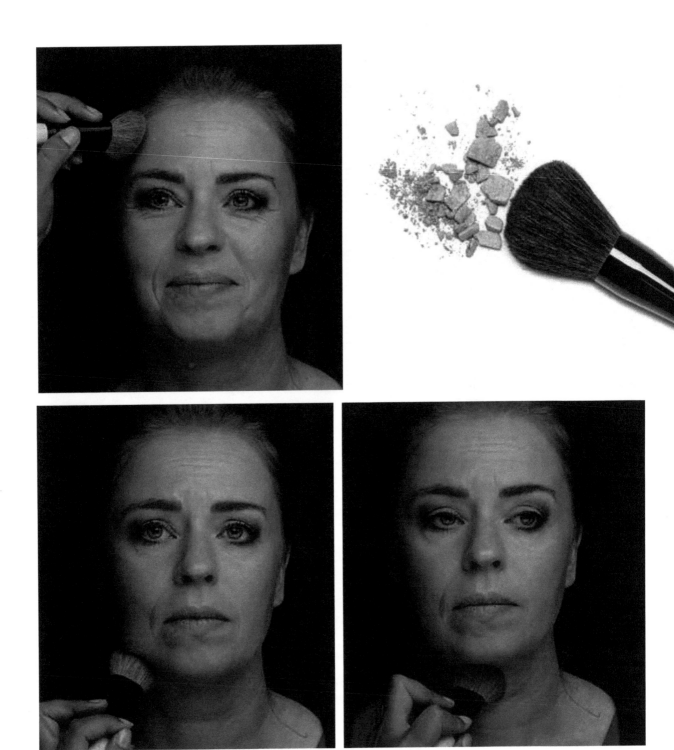

If you are concerned about a double chin you can create a small V just under the chin area.

Applying Blush

Once you've applied and blended your foundation and contour powder, you can add a little blush to bring your cheeks to life.

Blush is one of the few things a mature makeup application should never go without as it gives a flushed and healthy look to the skin, therefore making the face appear more youthful.

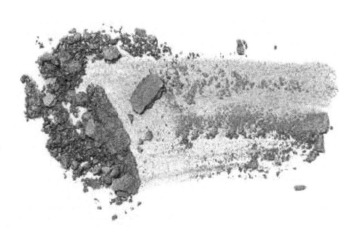

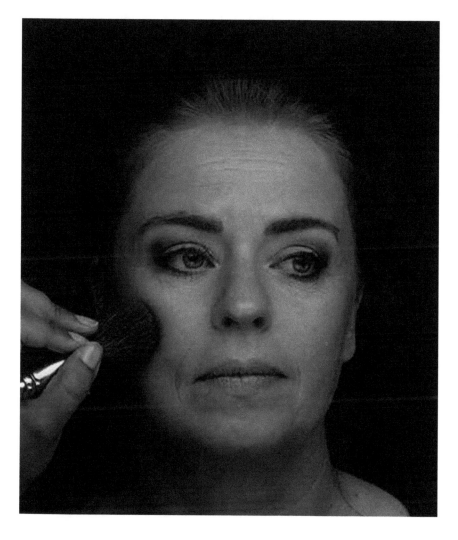

Using your blusher brush, sweep a light application of powder on the cheek in an upwards direction towards the temples – as opposed to the contouring colour which was applied under the cheek.

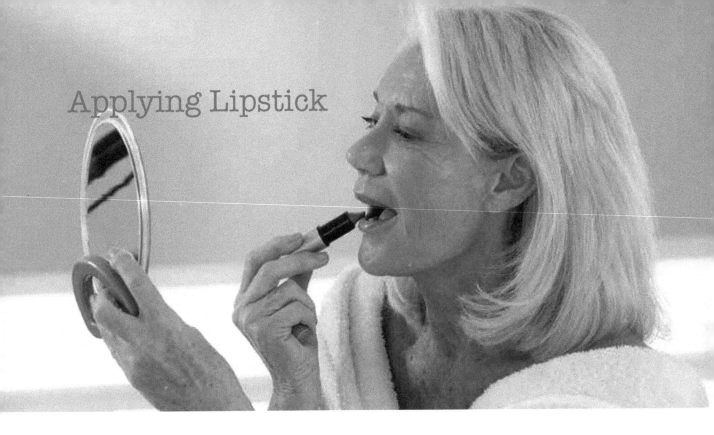

Applying Lipstick

Prepare the lips

For truly kissable lips it is important to lightly buff your lips to remove any dry skin. This gives your lipstick a smooth surface to which it can adhere and creates a smooth appearance. You can make a simple but effective sugar scrub as mentioned before, or alternately you can gently scrub your lips with a toothbrush in a small circular motion.

Line the lips

Apply a lip liner to the borders of your mouth, starting with the cupids bow (the two peaks at the top of the lip) and moving on to the middle of the lower lip.

By applying liner to these two areas first, it is easier to join up the outer edges of the lips to these two central points.

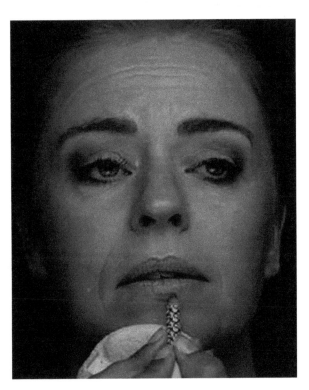

Fill the lips

Once you have created an outline to your lips, you can either fill the centre using your lip liner or your chosen lipstick. If you find that your lipstick comes off quickly, then filling in the with your lip liner prior to applying your lipstick will provide a base stain to your lips and add depth to the colour of the lipstick.

You can apply your lipstick straight from the tube, which will give a stronger colour, or with a lip brush. The latter will give your lipstick application a smoother finish, however you may need to apply a few coats to give the same intensity of colour that you would get from the lipstick direct.

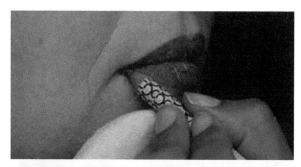

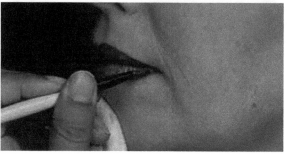

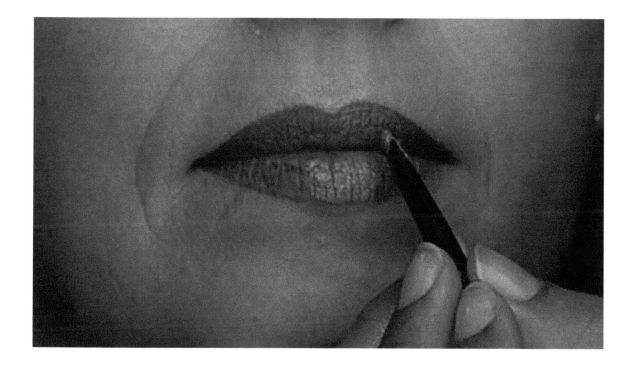

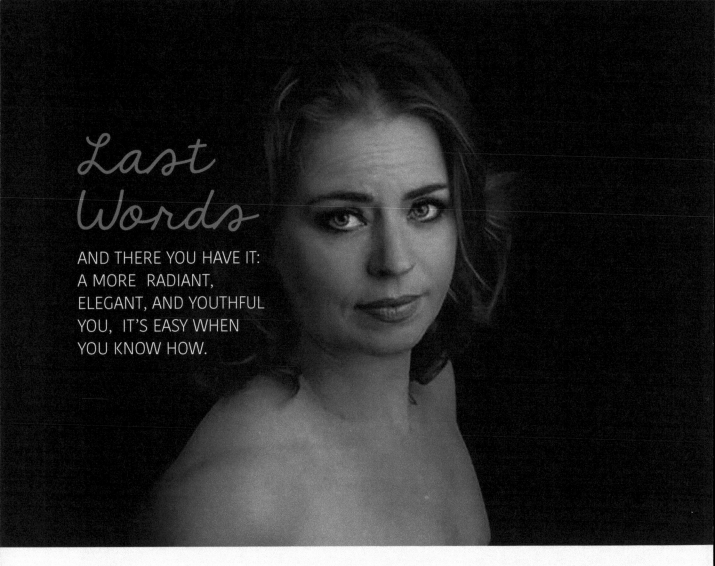

Last Words

AND THERE YOU HAVE IT:
A MORE RADIANT,
ELEGANT, AND YOUTHFUL
YOU, IT'S EASY WHEN
YOU KNOW HOW.

Many women are confused and frustrated when it comes to applying makeup, but with the right techniques, application and colour choices, anyone can transform their appearance to emphasise the beauty they already possess. So, instead of sticking to the same old makeup routine you have used for years, take a little time to learn how to highlight your finest features and draw attention away from your lines of experience.

A natural, complimentary application of makeup will not only help you look your best, but also make you feel confident and ready to face the world. You don't need to become a glamour puss, but the satisfaction of knowing that you look good is something that all women can experience and, with a few tricks of the trade, you can still look as vibrant as you did twenty years ago.

Your beauty grows with age as you show years of experience and wisdom on your face. While you should embrace the memories and appreciate the life you have lived, you can also learn how to hide the passage of time on your face and accentuate your best features. As Eartha Kitt once said, "Aging has a wonderful beauty and we should have respect for that."

CPSIA information can be obtained
at www.ICGtesting.com
Printed in the USA
LVHW081527250523
748065LV00017B/449